TOO MANY PEOPLE . . .

The small waiting room, save for the faint hissing of the heating system, was quiet when he walked in. The boy's mother was still in the chair. Her husband's arm, Allan noticed, was trembling while he grasped his wife's shoulders.

As he walked toward them he could see by their eyes that he was signalling his message. The woman turned away from him and, breaking into sobs, buried her face in the crook of her husband's arm. The man's face contorted as he struggled for composure.

Allan, now fighting himself against a surge of his emotions, spoke quietly, almost as if he wished they could not hear him. "We got him here as soon as possible and we did everything we could. . . . *Liar!* shot through his mind. "We were about to rush him to the operating room when his heart stopped. I'm sorry."

The man bent over and pressed his face to his wife's head. His shoulders shook. Allan wanted desperately to escape, to bolt out the door, to leave behind the grief that was building to an explosion. *That boy should be alive.*

. . . ARE DYING!

TRAUMA

TRAUMA

John J. Fried and John G. West, M.D.

PaperJacks LTD.

TORONTO   NEW YORK

PaperJacks

TRAUMA

PaperJacks LTD.

330 STEELCASE RD. E., MARKHAM, ONT. L3R 2M1
210 FIFTH AVE., NEW YORK, N.Y. 10010

Holt Rinehart and Winston edition published 1985

PaperJacks edition published February 1987

This is a work of fiction in its entirety. Any resemblance to actual people, places or events is purely coincidental.

ISBN 0-7701-0453-3

Across the country, hundreds of physicians, nurses, and lay support workers are working diligently to diminish the toll trauma takes on Americans. This novel is dedicated to their efforts.

Acknowledgments

Many people graciously gave of their time and expertise while we wrote this book. Medical advice came from Margie Murdock, R.N., B.S.N., Trauma Coordinator at the University of California, Irvine Medical Center; Donald L. Hicks, Vice-President of Development and Marketing, St. Joseph Hospital, Orange, California; Kevin Tremper, M.D., Ph.D., Acting Chairman of the Department of Anesthesiology and Assistant Professor of Anesthesiology, University of California, Irvine; Kenneth L. Mattox, M.D., Assistant Professor of Surgery, Baylor College of Medicine. Allan Martin gave us guidance on the legal issues, and Randy Cole helped keep the word processor running. Marilyn Cummings had many helpful suggestions for us as did Bob Heilig, Barbara Halligan, and Pat Siegel. Jan West, R.N., shared her expertise, and Chris Fried read and reread the manuscript with a sharp eye for inconsistencies and errors.

We are in particular debt to Michael Fisher of Praeger Scientific Publications, who recognized the potential in the story we wanted to tell and who took it upon himself to recommend the book to other professionals in his field in New York. Finally, we are grateful to Bobbi Mark of Holt, Rinehart and Winston for her encouragement and advice.

John J. Fried
Los Angeles, California

John G. West, M.D.
Orange, California

TRAUMA

1

"Dr. Kirk, Dr. Kirk," a soft voice said. The hand squeezed his left shoulder, at the same time gently rocking him. "Sorry to bother you, Dr. Kirk. The paramedics just brought someone in."

Allan Kirk looked up without comprehension toward the origin of the sound and saw a round face, its light-brown skin framed by black hair disheveled by the rush of ten hours in the emergency room. The smell of sweat filled the small room where he had been napping, but he was not sure now whether it came from him or from the woman who owned the face. Focusing, he saw she was the Filipino nurse working the emergency room with him.

"You all right, doctor?"

"Yes, sorry. Fine," he finally managed, rubbing the heels of his hands over his eyes. "Be right there."

As she turned to go, he groped for his watch on the small table next to him. He pulled it close to his face. Though the digital figures told him it was 3:06 A.M., it took him a few seconds to remember that it was now Sunday. He had been on duty for more than thirty hours.

He made his way through the door that led to the small

bathroom adjacent to the sleeping quarters Coit Hill Memorial Medical Center provided for doctors working the emergency room. He splashed water on his face and for a moment stared at himself in the mirror. At the age of thirty-four he had already finished five years of surgical training and was now in his second year of a fellowship at the University of California in San Francisco. Though he was far advanced in his career at the University, six weeks earlier he had begun moonlighting at various community hospitals around the county in order to finally sweep clean the slate of debts he had incurred to finance his medical education. But the seventy-two-hour weeks at the University—time he was dedicating to building a surgical division for the University that would specialize in treating trauma patients—coupled with his shifts at other hospitals, were taking a heavy toll. His naturally lean face looked drawn, even haggard. His eyes, which once had sparkled with curiosity and a fever to accomplish, seemed dull and almost obscured by the dark hollows around them. His hair, already highlighted by gray here and there, lay limp and lifeless on his head.

He moved from the bathroom into an adjoining room, really little more than an oversized closet. Most of the space was taken up by shelves full of surgical uniforms, masks, and paper booties. The minute floor area was dominated by a table cluttered with a coffee urn, mugs, a bottle of powdered cream, and an assortment of sweetening products. Wearily he scanned the shelves, looking for a set of old, worn greens, the sort he preferred because they were softer but fit tighter. He slipped his sockless feet back into the loafers he always wore so as not to waste time tying shoelaces, took a mug off the table, filled it three-quarters full with coffee, and then added four heaping spoons of sugar. He liked neither coffee nor sugar, but he needed the former to pry his mind out of sleep and the latter to give him quick energy.

As he entered the hospital's emergency room, he saw two paramedics hastily making for the exit and their van, parked just outside the doors. One of the men kept going but the other stopped when Allan called out.

"Hey, doc, you awake yet?" he kidded. "You look like one of our clients."

"I feel like it. What have you dragged me out of bed for?"

"College kid, some buddies, and their girls had been eating pizza and drinking beer, then went joyriding on their motorcycles. The others saw a red light he sort of missed. He went through it and got broadsided by a pickup. The gal riding with him was killed. He was knocked out but started coming around on the run in here. Still confused though, kept calling for his mama."

"Vital signs?"

"Seemed okay out there. Blood pressure was 110/70 and his pulse was a hundred-ten."

"What's the timing on the kid?"

"He got creamed about three o'clock. We had just finished another call in the area, so we got right to him."

Allan glanced at his watch. It was 3:10. If the biker was seriously injured, he had to move quickly.

The paramedic who had gone out to the van came back to the door. "Come on, Jack, we got a cardiac call, let's move."

"We gotta go, doc. The kid's in Resuscitation Room B." Allan nodded to the paramedic and, still trying to shake the fatigue from his body, forced himself to trot toward the room.

On a bed just inside the door lay a muscular young man, dressed in jeans and a University of California sweatshirt with sleeves cut off at the shoulders. He looked about eighteen or nineteen. The biker's muscles bulged as, trying to get up, he deliriously grabbed at the gurney's raised side rails. He was yelling obscenities, demanding to be told where he was, and still crying plaintively for his mother. The boys who are hurt, Allan thought as he moved quickly to the side of the bed, always cry for their mothers.

The biker's yells told Allan that nothing was obstructing his air passages and that he was able to breathe on his own. Allan put his hand on the boy's wrist. He could feel the pulse, but it was alarmingly fast. The boy's face was pale. Small beads of sweat were forming on his forehead. Blood vessels constricting to keep the blood pressure up, Allan noted. He's going into shock.

The sound of shuffling paper caught Allan's attention. He looked up and saw the Filipino nurse, Esperanza Gomez, sitting on a stool in a corner of the room, busily filling out one of the countless forms she would have to complete for the boy's medical records. She was working at her task diligently, as if it were one of the most crucial medical procedures she could perform.

Allan made a strong and successful effort to fight off his usual impatience. "Would you mind putting that aside for a moment and taking his blood pressure?"

"Oh, doctor, it's okay. I just checked it before you came in. Pressure was 100/60. Pulse one-twenty per minute. Respiration okay."

"Get the pressure again," Allan said, determined to maintain his composure, even though she was not up to date on her information and didn't seem bothered by the fact. Her equanimity, he was sure, was rooted less in indifference than in inexperience: she could not appreciate the urgency of the moment.

"Get a cut-down tray, stat," he said, after she had taken the blood pressure again. He put his hands on the boy's head. There was a nasty scrape starting at the temple and running down the side of his face.

"Hey, kid," Allan said, hoping to get a response that would tell him something about the boy's mental condition. "Tell me your name. What's your name?"

The boy mumbled incoherently. "Ma" was the only word Allan could make out. Though the biker's pupils looked normal, he made a mental note to have a neurosurgeon come in later to check on the boy, and he went on with the exam. He ran his hands from the boy's neck down to the sides of his rib cage. The ribs on the left felt normal. But on the lower right he felt the sharp edges of broken ribs rubbing against each other. Allan's hands continued downward. He pushed down gently on the belly. He could feel the muscles contract on the upper right-hand side, over the liver. The boy groaned and tried to push him away. Allan resisted the move and pushed in on the pelvic bones. The boy cried out again.

"Sorry, kid," Allan said. "Not trying to hurt you. I have to find out what's wrong if we're going to help you." At a minimum, Allan said to himself, this guy has traumatic injury to the liver, pelvic fractures, and multiple rib fractures.

Allan looked up to see if the nurse had gone to get the instruments he had requested. To his amazement, she had not moved. She met his gaze wide-eyed.

He started to bark, but stopped. "What are you waiting for?" he said with measured control.

"Doctor, I am sorry. We don't have a cut-down tray here. I must send down to central supply for it."

He glanced up at the clock on the wall. It read 3:14. Only a few minutes had gone by since he had stepped into the room, but Allan felt a wave of apprehension sweep over him. He was convinced the boy was bleeding internally. Allan always preached to medical students and interns that if a grievously injured patient was to be saved, internal bleeding had to be controlled within the first hour the patient had been hurt. Since the boy had been injured at three, fourteen minutes of his "Golden Hour" had already passed. In the next forty-six minutes we have a lot to do, Allan told himself while looking at the willing but confused nurse, and it doesn't look as if I'm going to get much help here.

He took a long, deep breath, held it, and let it out slowly. "Okay," he said. "Never mind the cut-down, get an IV set up in his right arm. I'll use a fourteen-gauge intracut catheter and a liter of Ringer's lactate on the left arm."

She started to move. "Before you do that," Allan said, stopping her in her tracks, "get on the intercom and have the receptionist get the nursing supervisor, the lab tech, and someone for a portable X ray down here. Stat."

As she turned to go to the phone, Allan reached for the large bandage scissors he had attached to his greens with a safety pin. With quick motions, he cut off the biker's shirt, pants, and underpants. The boy lay naked now except for scuffed cowboy boots that reached well upward toward his knees. He moved to the end of the table and grasped the heel of the boot on the biker's left foot. He started to pull the boot, but immediately realized, with some terror, that the boot was wobbling abnormally on the leg. Bending closer to the limb, Allan could see a gaping wound just below the top of the boot. Tilting the boot ever so slightly, Allan spotted fragments of bone showing through the wound.

With a chill he realized that he had been a fool for hurrying to pull the boot without bothering to check for bone damage. If he had persisted he would have amputated the boy's lower leg.

Gomez, he now saw with some satisfaction, had set up the IV he had asked for, but neither the lab nor the X-ray technicians had yet materialized.

"I need him typed and crossed for eight units of blood. What's taking the lab tech so long?" he muttered. "What the hell is wrong with this place?"

"Dr. Kirk, there is nothing wrong with this hospital, I can assure you. The X-ray technician is busy in the ICU. The other techs are also busy and can't be in two places at once. They'll be here as soon as possible." The speaker was Gloria Cluny, the night nursing supervisor, a woman he had met in his first round of duty at the hospital a week earlier. Great, he said to himself, not only do I have an inexperienced nurse to work with, but now I'm going to have to deal with a passive-aggressive nut who'll give me grief instead of help.

Cluny was a stout, matronly woman who viewed the world through flat brown eyes and rimless glasses. Though she was probably in her early fifties, the glasses and the way she wore her hair—tightly pulled back into a small knot at the back of her head—made her look older. This nurse, Allan had heard from some of the other emergency-room doctors who had worked shifts at Coit Hill, was a stickler for rules and regulations. And rules and regulations, he knew, were only likely to become obstacles during the countdown leading to the final few minutes that would determine whether his patient would live or die.

But Allan, knowing all this and disliking her for it, was still determined to be civil toward her. If he had any chance of saving the boy's life, he would need every bit of cooperation he could get out of her. She had made her entrance at 3:20. Only forty minutes of the biker's Golden Hour remained.

Allan forced himself to smile, hoping that the smile had an appropriately sheepish quality to it. "Sorry. I'm sure the techs are doing their best. But I'm worried about this kid, he may bleed out on us. I need a surgeon and an anesthesiologist in here. Would you please call them? Oh, and could you get an O.R. open?"

She regarded him coldly. "Certainly, doctor." She turned on her heels to leave the room, but stopped. "Perhaps you'd like to talk to the boy's parents now?"

"Crap! Are they here already?" As long as he had worked in emergency rooms and as often as he had handled trauma cases, he had always found it hard to talk to relatives of badly injured patients, particularly the parents of young people. The way they looked at him made him feel that superhuman efforts were expected of him. And if the patient had died, their gazes always accused him of having failed where he might have succeeded. Now, convinced that the boy had massive internal injuries, and unsure when a surgeon would arrive, Allan felt an even stronger reluctance tugging at him.

Repressing his feelings, Allan walked quickly out of the emergency room to a door that bore a Private sign. He took a deep breath, took hold of the handle, pulled, and went in. A woman was sitting in one of the two easy chairs in the room. Strands of gray hair peeked out from under a rain hat she had obviously pulled on in a hurry. She was wearing an old raincoat, the kind San Franciscans keep in the front closet to wear when they have to dash out with the garbage on a rainy night. Allan couldn't see her face because her head was bent, her eyes riveted on her cupped hands resting in her lap. A man stood behind her, one hand on her shoulder. He was tall and gaunt. His face was shadowed by the nighttime stubble. His eyes widened as Allan came farther into the room.

The woman, who had not heard Allan come in, looked up now too, alerted by the shift in her husband's hand. She sprang to her feet. "My boy, doctor?" she pleaded. "Is he all right? Please tell me he's all right. The nurse who called said—"

"Say it's a mistake, doc?" the man interrupted. "Greg is supposed to be over in Berkeley. He's in school there. He wouldn't be over here. It's not Greg, is it?"

Allan led the woman back to her chair. He looked at the man, then back at her. His heart was pounding and the insides of his mouth had turned to chalk. "No, I'm sorry, it's not a mistake." He felt his tongue sticking to the roof of his mouth as he spoke. He thought he must be mumbling incomprehensibly. "Greg and his girl friend were over on this side of the Bay. They were riding back to the University when they were broadsided by a small truck. . . ."

The first sounds of the woman's sobbing interrupted him. Greg's father was breathing deeply, audibly, struggling to maintain control. An absurd thought crossed Allan's mind as he listened to the man's chest: He's a heavy smoker. He should quit. "Ma'am," he said, making an effort to sound as reassuring and as soothing as possible, "We're doing everything we can. I'll try to keep you posted."

Allan made for the door. The boy's father caught up with him. "He's our only child, doctor," he said. Allan thought the man was trying to think of something else to add, but nothing else came. Allan nodded and walked out.

He ran back into the emergency room and almost collided with a lab technician carrying a basket with the tools needed to draw blood. A woman pushing a portable X-ray machine was right behind the technician. Hoping to hurry things along, Allan helped her propel the cumbersome piece of equipment into the resuscitation room.

"Dr. Kirk!" Gomez called to him. "Patient's blood pressure just dropped to 60/40."

"This kid is bleeding badly inside, no question," Allan said. "He should be in the O.R. by now, and we're still screwing around with IVs." He stopped himself. "He is going to need all the fluids he can get if he's going to stay alive long enough to get a surgeon in here."

Allan turned to the lab tech. "I'm going to need blood in here as quickly as possible."

He turned back to Gomez. "We're not going to get all the fluids and blood he needs into him with just the two IVs we have going. Get me a scalpel and some sterile IV tubing."

"What kind of catheter to go with tubing, doctor?"

"Never mind the catheter, we'll put the tubing right into the saphenous vein in the right ankle."

While he slipped on gloves, the nurse poured a liberal dose of an antiseptic solution on the ankle. Allan followed with an anesthetic and, almost without pausing, grabbed a scalpel. He cut through the pale skin with a long, smooth slice and then with two or three softer strokes cut through the yellow globules of fat beneath the surface until he could see the soft, white fibery surface of the vein he was after. With a deliberate motion he nicked the vein. He slipped a clamp beneath the vessel to prevent blood from pouring out and obscuring his vision. Gomez handed him the IV tubing and he gently threaded it, through the nick he had made, into the center of the vein. The nurse connected the other side of the tubing to a bottle of Ringer's lactate and opened the valve wide to allow the fluid to pour into the biker's body. The nurse scurried to remeasure his blood pressure. "It's back to 100/60, doctor."

"Okay for now. Keep the IVs wide open." He turned and called out through the door that had been left open by the technicians. "Where do we stand on getting a surgeon in here?"

"Dr. Weiss is on first call, but his answering service can't find him," Cluny called back.

"All right, call the next one," he said out loud, "And call the bank and get some blood down here." Allan looked at the clock—four more minutes had elapsed—then back at the boy lying naked on the gurney. Only semiconscious, he tossed his head back and forth and mumbled obscenities. Allan put his stethoscope to the boy's chest. He had a hard time hearing breathing sounds from the right lung, a sign that the boy was bleeding into that side of the chest. He ran his hands over the biker's belly. There was more tenderness now, much of it spreading to his lower abdomen. Allan glanced at the clock. It was almost half past the hour. He estimated the boy had another thirty-five minutes to live. From the clock his glance fell on the lab technician who had silently reentered the room. The man's face was gloomy.

"That was fast," Allan said. "Have you typed and crossed him already?"

"Yeah. Doctor, I thought I should tell you myself that we have a problem with the blood," the technician said quietly. "The kid is O positive. But Dr. Harper used up our entire supply of O positive, plus all we could get from the Red Cross, for an aneurysm that he had to resect about four hours ago. All I have is what I brought with me. Two units of universal-donor O-negative blood."

"Shit!" Allan exploded. "All right, thanks. Get those two units hung." He leaned so he could look past the technician. "We've got to get someone in here," he called out to Cluny. "Where do you stand on the on-call surgeon?"

"I've called Dr. Goodenouw but he's on vacation. He's got someone covering for him, but that man does not have staff privileges here." Allan thought he could sense frustration creeping into Cluny's voice.

"We're running out of time! Who is responsible for the on-call schedule?"

"Dr. Harper, the chief of staff. But he's not on call. And besides he was here till one o'clock with the ruptured aneurysm."

"Get him on the line and I'll talk to him and that will at least save a step."

As Cluny dialed the number, Allan walked to the counter. Through window a few feet behind the counter he could see the boy's father pacing, smoking a cigarette. Cluny spoke quickly into the receiver, then handed it to Allan. He introduced himself.

"Listen, Kirk," Harper interrupted. "I was down there well past midnight. Now what do you have that's so all-fired important that they gotta wake me up at three-thirty in the morning?"

Allan reminded himself to stay cool and described the biker's injuries, his efforts to keep the boy's blood pressure up, the lack of blood at the hospital. The minute he uttered the information about the blood he knew he had made a strategic mistake.

"Dr. Kirk," Harper interrupted. "It sounds to me as if you have somebody there with irreparable injuries. I've covered that E.R., young man, and I've seen a thousand cases like that. I'm sorry, but it's not worthwhile my coming in. There are just some cases that are beyond repair. You can't save everybody."

Allan turned from the counter. The door to the emergency room opened. The boy's father tentatively stuck his head into the room and looked around. Allan, afraid he would see his son without being prepared for the sight, motioned to him to stop. The father began walking toward him.

Allan pressed the phone closer to his face. "Dr. Harper," he said quickly. "The boy is salvageable if we can stop his internal bleeding before another twenty-five or thirty minutes get by."

"Listen, kid," Harper said, putting emphasis on the "kid." "That boy is as good as dead even if Christ himself were to rush down and operate. And you just told me you haven't even got enough blood in the bank to warrant going in."

Allan turned around so that he was facing away from the boy's father who stood at a distance, waiting.

"The Red Cross says they can get us a dozen units," he lied.

"I seriously doubt that. And even if they could, you'd just be pouring them down a sieve. Learn when to give up, doctor. Go back and get some sleep and let me do the same."

Allan could sense that Harper was about to hang up without even the benefit of a goodnight. "Harper!" he hissed into the phone, trying to keep his voice at a whisper. "I guarantee you that I can keep the boy alive until you can get here. I'll take responsibility for that. But if you don't leave now and he dies, then it's your responsibility and I'll make damn sure that you answer for the death." Allan could feel himself sweating, the audacity of the words he had just blurted out coming home to him.

Harper's breath came at him over the phone. "All right," the physician finally said. "I'm coming in. It'll take me twenty minutes. But that boy better be breathing when I get there."

Allan, shaking, put down the phone and hurried to the biker's father. Allan put his hand on the man's elbow and gently guided him out the door.

"I've just talked to a surgeon," Allan said, while the man lifted a cigarette to his mouth with a badly trembling hand. "He'll be here in twenty minutes."

"He needs surgery?" his voice broke. "Greg needs an operation?"

"Yes. But it's no cause for alarm. Once we get him into the operating room he's as good as on his way home. Believe me."

The man looked at him, his eyes shimmering. He raised the hand carrying the cigarette and wiped at his eyes with the knuckle of his index finger. "Doc, if that boy dies . . . I don't know what we're gonna do. . . ."

"We're doing all we can," Allan answered. "Come on, help us out. Go back and wait with your wife."

Allan bolted back into the emergency room and to the biker.

Just as he reached his bedside the X-ray technician came running in with the X rays of the boy's chest. She slapped them onto the viewing box and flipped on the light switch for Allan. Allan scanned the films quickly. They confirmed his suspicion that there was blood in the right side of the boy's chest.

"We're going to have to put in a chest tube," he said to Gomez. "Get me a thirty-six-French chest tube and set up a pleurovac. Stat."

The nurse fidgeted. "We don't have a thirty-six-French." She hesitated.

"All right, all right. Just give me whatever selection of tubes you've got. I'll pick what I need. Let's get going. And, while you're at it, get me gloves, Betadine, a scalpel, a ten-cubic-centimeter syringe, Xylocaine, a suture set with O silk on a large needle, and two-inch tape. Get going."

Gomez scurried back with the tray. Allan grabbed the gloves and worked his fingers into them, watching as she painted antiseptic on the area where the tube would enter the boy's body.

As soon as she was done, Allan located the fifth rib and pushed the syringe filled with the anesthetic into the area. Almost without stopping he seized the scalpel and made a half-inch incision, put down the scalpel, grabbed for a clamp, and used it to spread open the cut he had made. Air rushed out of the opening, followed by a stream of blood. He pulled out the clamp, put his finger into the wound and twisted the digit to make sure the lung was not stuck to the chest wall. Satisfied it was not, he took the 28-French tube and pushed it deep into the chest. A gusher of blood came spurting out at him, splattering his and the nurse's uniform and staining the sheets of the gurney. He allowed himself a smile but at the same time caught the covert surprised look Gomez had given him.

"We hit a gusher," he explained, speaking as if he were addressing a group of his students. "That's our sign that we've made the right decision, that there has been hemorrhaging endangering the patient. There is nothing more upsetting than to shove in a chest tube, to do something so brutal to a patient, and have just a few drops of blood come dripping out. Gonna make it nurse-proof now," he continued. "Nothing worse than to put one of these in and have some nurse on the floor the first night out of school come along and pull it out." As he taped he continued the monologue. "They're going to be able to hang this guy from the ceiling by the tube and it isn't going to come out. Okay, let's get a repeat chest X ray to make sure we haven't pushed the tube through the diaphragm and into the liver."

Allan looked at the clock: 3:36 A.M. Another six minutes had elapsed. With the chest tube he had drained off escaped blood, thereby allowing the lung to reexpand, but the main threat was still the bleeding in the abdomen. The boy was down to the last fifteen minutes or so during which it would still be possible to save his life by controlling the bleeding.

Allan ran for the door. "We're going to need more blood," he called out in Cluny's general direction. "Give the blood bank downtown another try. If they don't have anything, put out a call to police headquarters and the fire-department dispatcher. Maybe we can get some pints out of people on duty now." He started to go back into the room. Remembering that the boy had been knocked out by the accident, recalling the bruise on his temple and his confused mumblings, Allan turned around. "Then see if you can get a neurosurgeon in here too."

"We can't get one if we haven't done the CAT scan," Cluny answered. "We have two neurosurgeons on staff and neither of them will come if a CAT scan hasn't been done."

"Okay. Let's get it done."

"We can't. The technician is home. It'll take her forty-five minutes to get here and then another half hour to get the machine warmed up enough. If you phone either of the neurosurgeons on call and give them CAT-scan results more than two hours after the patient has been brought in, they'll tell you that if he has made it this far without a neuro consult, he'll make it until they get in in the morning, do their scheduled surgeries, and have time to see him during rounds. I know the routine. It's happened before." Cluny stopped. "How about an orthopedic surgeon?" she asked, as if trying to make up for her inability to get a neurosurgeon in.

"Hell, no, he's the one guy we gotta keep out of here. Call in an orthopod, and he'll just foul everything up by ordering a lot of unnecessary tests. I'll just splint the fracture. Once we get the kid stabilized in the O.R., then we'll let the orthopod in. If you can't get a neurosurgeon in as well, I'll settle for Harper getting here on time. That's all the kid needs now."

He turned his attention back to the boy. His skin was the color of chalk. Sweat was pouring off his naked body. "Let's get his blood pressure again," he told Gomez.

"His blood pressure is back down to eighty, doctor, and his pulse back to one-twenty," she announced, trying to make herself helpful.

While he had been talking to the boy's father, either Gomez or Cluny had placed a catheter in the boy's bladder. Allan looked at the bag at the other end of the tube. There was only a small collection of urine at its bottom.

"How long ago did you empty the urine collecting bag?" Allan asked.

"We cathed him for two hundred cc's ten minutes ago and he has not made urine since that time, doctor," Gomez answered in a whisper.

Allan could feel his shirt sticking to his wet back. His eyes were burning, his neck was stiffening up on him, his legs were lead. The biker's small urine output, he concluded, meant the kidneys had shut down as shock was continuing its attack. The vessels that were pouring blood into the boy's belly had to be sewn up. And yet, the clock told him it would be at least another ten, perhaps twelve, minutes before Harper made it through the doors. Allan again felt desperation set in. By the time they got the kid under anesthesia . . .

He stopped in mid-thought, now truly frightened. Fighting to remain calm, he jogged back to the emergency-room counter where Cluny was now coolly making out another sheaf of forms. "Miss Cluny, have you called in an anesthesiologist?"

She finished a word she was writing, then looked up at him. "No, Dr. Kirk, there is not much sense in doing so until Dr. Harper gets here. At this hospital the anesthesiologist is not called until the surgeon has seen the patient and has decided to take him to the operating room."

"Miss Cluny, Dr. Harper has as much as agreed to operate on

the boy. Would you please get whatever gasser is on call in here. Please!"

"I'm sorry, doctor, but those are the rules. I will certainly not preempt Dr. Harper."

Without uttering another word, Allan pushed aside the small swinging door that gave access to the area behind the counter and made for the telephone. Just above it was the on-call list. He ran down the names and the listings of specialists until he found the anesthesiologist. With now barely restrained fury he punched at the phone buttons. When the anesthesiologist answered, Allan, in a rush of words, explained the situation and virtually ordered the man in.

"Kirk, I've never heard of you, so I'm assuming you are new around there. So let me fill you in, just in case no one else has—"

"If you're going to tell me about a surgeon having to call you in, Dr. Harper is coming in. I'm sure he's going to take the boy to the O.R. Look, we haven't got a lot of time. Minutes . . ."

"Never mind the drama. I don't know how you got Harper to come in. But I'm not about to rush in in the middle of the night on your word. I've got a full schedule in the morning."

"Doctor, your responsibility . . ."

"Hey, don't lecture me about responsibility. I bet that kid isn't doing more than bleeding from a pelvic fracture and the abdominal tenderness may be nothing more than a result of the fractured ribs. It'll hold. I bet you haven't even done a peritoneal lavage."

"It's not necessary."

"It is to me. How do I know he's bleeding into the abdomen? You call me back when the lavage's done and if Harper isn't there by that time, I'll think about coming in." And with that he hung up.

Allan slowly put down the receiver and glanced at his watch. It blinked 3:52 at him. He felt as if he had been working here a lifetime. The muscles of his lower back were screaming in pain, his legs felt rubbery. His arms felt heavy, pulled on, as if gravity itself had made them a test case for its power.

He dragged himself back to the biker's side. The skirmishes over the cut-down and the chest tube were only just behind him and now he would have to tap the biker's abdomen for the telltale signs of a massive internal hemorrhage. But he was determined to have the anesthesiologist come in. And if he did not do the lavage, he would not be able to persuade the man to come in.

He approached Gomez and, hoping she would know what he was talking about, asked her for a peritoneal lavage tray. "We've never used one in here at night," she answered. It was a roundabout way of saying, he was convinced, that she had no idea what a lavage tray was. But before he had a chance to go on, Cluny materialized next to them.

"Do me a favor," he said, determined to stay civilized, but feeling that he was only barely in control of himself, because he could detect a tinge of panic in his own voice. "Go to central supply and see if you can find a lavage tray." In two minutes she was back, carrying the tray. Allan thought he would weep for joy.

While he wiggled into yet another set of sterile gloves, Gomez first shaved the biker's abdomen an inch below the belly button, then swabbed it with a strong antiseptic. Quickly, Allan made a small cut into the prepped skin. He grabbed for a rigid plastic tube with a knifelike structure at one end, a large rounded plastic knob on the other. He put the knife to the cut at a forty-five-degree angle, aiming it toward the pelvis. As Allan pushed on the round knob, the knife cut down into the abdominal cavity. He had only pushed about a quarter of an inch when the biker began to groan and grunt, tensing his muscles. Allan didn't let up. With steady and firm pressure he punctured the abdominal wall. The tube slid slightly inward.

He guided it forward another six or eight inches. A squirt of blood flew high into the air. For the briefest of moments Allan was terrified, concerned, as he always was when he performed a lavage, that he might have hit the aorta or another major vessel. But the gushing slowed to a gentle bubbling and then a trickle. He had tapped into the large pool of loose blood that was, just as he had believed, accumulating in the abdominal cavity. With a quick flick of the hand, he pulled the catheter out of the abdomen. The boy groaned heavily and tried to twist on to his side.

There was a strange silence in the emergency room. He looked up to see Gomez and Cluny looking at him, something approaching respect in their eyes. He walked back to the counter, found the anesthesiologist's number and dialed. The others watched as he talked into the phone, then hung up the receiver.

"His answering service picked up," he said in response to the unspoken question. "They said he left orders not to be disturbed unless the on-call surgeon wants to speak to him."

He walked back to the boy's side. "If Harper is not here in the next five minutes . . ." In his mind he was already seeing himself signing the boy's death certificate. What would he put on the line that called for his opinion on the cause of death? "Patient expired due to medical indifference"? Or, "Patient died because surgeons don't know shit about trauma"?

What would happen, he wondered, if he tried to operate on the boy himself. He turned to Cluny, who had joined him in the treatment room. "I'm going to take him in to the O.R.," he said with a determination he hoped would sway her.

"Dr. Kirk, why didn't you say you had O.R. privileges here?" Her voice was icy.

"I don't . . . ," Allan stammered.

"Then what on earth are you talking about? I certainly will not open the O.R. for someone who has no standing on the staff here. What an idea!" She cast him a haughty look, then relented. "Be patient, Dr. Kirk. It's almost four. Dr. Harper will be here within five minutes."

Allan ignored the remark. "Can we transfer him to the University? There are provisions for that."

"We could, except that the County Health Department rules clearly state that no patient whose vital signs are as unstable as that boy's can be transferred. I'm sorry, but I won't make or authorize a call to the paramedics to transport him."

He pounded the small table that held the bloodied instruments he had used for the chest tube and the lavage. This fuckin' system, he said to himself, as he looked around in desperation. I can't get anyone to come in because no one cares about cases like this. I can't fuckin' operate because I haven't got privileges. I can't send him to the University because he can't get up and jog over there by himself.

"Doctor!" Gomez yelled. "His blood pressure is down, 40/0!"

Allan's first impulse was to order some more blood, but he stopped himself as he remembered they had already used every unit the hospital had available, that there had been no response yet to their calls to outside agencies. The boy's parents? Even if they were both the right blood type, that would mean only two pints, much less than he needed. Allan said nothing, turned on his heels, and rushed out of the emergency room and into the parking lot. His five-year-old Chevy gleamed a garish unnatural color under the high-intensity yellow lights that had been installed for nighttime safety. In a dozen strides he was at the trunk. He opened it, reached into a steel container marked CHC in large, bold, red letters, and took out a box of twelve plastic packets, each containing a creamy liquid.

He slammed shut the trunk and ran back to the emergency room. Gomez and Cluny were at the biker's side, furiously adjusting the valves on the IVs that had been allowing Ringer's lactate into the body.

"Forget that shit!" he yelled. "That's just sugar water, goddamnit. He needs something that's going to take oxygen to his tissues."

The boy's breathing was now coming in heavy, body-wracking rales. Abruptly, Allan reached for one of the Ringer's lactate bottles, disconnected it from the clear plastic tubing, and replaced it with one of the plastic bags he had retrieved from the car. After he had repeated the procedure with another IV, he took hold of one of the new bags and squeezed on it with one hand and grappled for the boy's wrist with the other. As he squeezed the bag, he could feel the boy's pulse grow stronger and slower.

"Blood pressure?" he asked.

"Moving up, doctor," Gomez replied, "80/60."

For a second Allan allowed himself to relax. Maybe the kid will make it, he said to himself, maybe Harper will walk in, right now. He looked down at the boy's face and focused on the dark bruise on the side of his face.

"Damnit," he said to no one in particular. "CAT scan or no CAT scan, I'm calling a neurosurgeon." He turned to Cluny and pointed to the two other bags he had brought in. "Pump these other units in when that one's done."

Cluny, who had watched him suspiciously when he returned from his car with his bags, made no move to obey him. "I have no idea what is in those bags, doctor. Unless you tell me, I will not be a party to injecting . . ."

Allan glared at her. He didn't know whether to go to the phone as he had planned or to stay in the room and see to the bags himself.

The dilemma was cut short by the shrill whistle that tore through the otherwise still resuscitation room. Gomez shouted, "Cardiac arrest!"

Allan looked at the cardiac monitor, saw the flat line, and immediately swung into action. The nurse started to run for the defibrillator, the machine that could shock the heart back into action.

"Never mind that," Allan shouted, anticipating her move. "We're going in. Get some Betadine on his chest."

Gomez poured the sterilizing liquid on the boy's chest. Allan grabbed a scalpel off the table, jabbed into the chest between the fourth and fifth ribs and, in a hard, steady motion, pulled the knife straight across and downward until the blade cut into the sheet beneath the boy's body. With two fingers he easily spread the exposed chest muscle, tearing the fibers that held it together. He picked up the scalpel again, this time to cut into the muscle between the ribs. With two more fast strokes the chest was completely open. He started to ask for a rib spreader. But knowing ahead of time what the answer would be, he stopped and instead pushed three fingers from each hand into the hole he had cut, and, using all his strength, spread apart the ribs.

Straining hard now, he pushed his right hand into the chest, almost immediately feeling the moist, warm pericardium, the sac containing the heart. The organ was twitching weakly, its efforts to continue beating more like weak shudders.

Allan squeezed the organ and felt it give easily. "It hasn't got a drop of blood in it," he said, then shouted: "Goddamnit! Gomez! Hang one of the bags, fast!"

Wide-eyed with fear because she was caught between Allan and a staring Cluny, Gomez nevertheless moved to follow his orders.

Allan squeezed the heart rhythmically, squeezing and releasing at what he estimated to be eighty to ninety beats a minute. There was no response. To test the heart, he eased his grip. The organ lay dead in his hands.

He began to squeeze again, trying, despite his agony, to ignore a developing and searing pain first in his forearm muscles, which were bearing the brunt of his squeezing action, then on his wrist, which was being cut again and again by the sharp ribs.

Cluny looked into the boy's eyes. "The pupils are fixed and dilated, doctor."

Allan slumped and slowly took his hand out of the biker's chest. He looked up. Standing at the door watching was an older man, fury etched into every portion of his face. Allan knew it was Harper.

"Doctor," Allan began, but stopped. Harper looked at him, shook his head in slow disgust, and, putting his raincoat back on, walked briskly away.

Neither Cluny nor Gomez looked at Allan. The receptionist, who had come out from behind her desk to watch what was obviously the final drama, moved back to her station. Gomez busied herself pulling out the various IV needles and draining tubes out of the boy's body, then covered his body with the urine-and blood-stained sheet. Cluny began to gather the scalpels and other assorted instruments and to dump them into a porcelain tray.

Allan looked out the double glass doors and saw that dawn was breaking. He felt anesthetized. He knew only that he wanted to get out, to come to grips with what had happened, to give his mind a chance to clear. To stop trembling.

Gomez's voice reached him. "The family, doctor? Are you going to talk to them?"

What am I going to do? he asked himself, fear washing coldly over him. Though he always felt remorse when he lost a patient, usually the feeling did not assault him fully until hours or even days had passed. But now the feeling came on him immediately. Should he have transferred the boy faster? Should he have raised more hell to get a surgeon in? How could he face these people?

He went to the sink in the resuscitation room and poured

cold water over his face and head. Slowly, stalling for time, he wiped his face and hands dry, then, irrationally, tucked his shirt into his pants. Maybe I can take one of the nurses in with me, he thought wildly, or maybe one of the social workers has come in early and she could talk to them.

The small waiting room, save for the faint hissing of the heating system, was quiet when he walked in. The boy's mother was still in the chair. Her husband's arm, Allan noticed, was trembling while he grasped his wife's shoulders.

As he walked toward them he could see by their eyes that he was signaling his message. The woman turned away from him and, breaking into sobs, buried her face in the crook of her husband's arm. The man's face contorted as he struggled for composure.

Allan, now fighting himself against a surge of his emotions, spoke quietly, almost as if he wished they could not hear him. "We got him here as soon as possible and we did everything we could. . . ." *Liar!* shot through his mind. "We were about to rush him to the operating room when his heart stopped. I'm sorry."

The man bent over and pressed his face to his wife's head. His shoulders shook. Allan wanted desperately to escape, to bolt out the door, to leave behind the grief that was building to an explosion. *That boy should be alive.* The thought ran through his mind, an endless refrain. His hands grew cold and wet. A gnawing pain began to eat away at his stomach. He wanted to stand up and scream, "Your son is dead! Your son is dead and this hospital with its doctors who don't care is responsible."

The woman looked at Allan, her face red and streaked by tears. "It's not Greg!" she screamed as she stood and took two steps toward Allan. "It's not my Greg. It's not. He's nineteen. My God, he's nineteen!" The husband shrank back. With a plea on his face he turned to Allan.

Allan put his hands on her shoulders and guided her back to the chair, then eased her into it. "I'll send a nurse in with something to help you," Allan said, incapable of finding anything else to say.

"I don't want anything," the woman cried. "I want my Greg back."

"Can we see him, doc?" the man asked.

Allan stopped and turned back. "Of course. But give the nurses a few minutes to clean up." Allan again headed for the door.

"Doc? His things?"

Allan led them to the emergency room's counter. The clerk had already put the boy's wallet, a bracelet he had been wearing on one wrist, and a necklace he had had around his neck in a plain brown paper bag. With a wan smile she handed the package to Greg's mother, who clutched it to her chest.

"We'll let you know when you can see him," the clerk said gently. "Why don't you wait in the hall for a few moments?"

Allan looked after them as they slowly made their way to the emergency-room door. When they were out of sight he took a last look around. Gomez was gone, but Cluny was still occupied cleaning the resuscitation room where they had worked on the boy. Allan looked past her, focusing first on the boy's face, then his naked, pale body. It was a death, something told him, that would haunt him, that he would not leave unchallenged. He turned and made for the parking lot and his car.

Cluny watched him for the entire time it took him to reach the emergency-room doors, wait for them to open automatically, and then pass through them. When he was out of sight she reached up, disconnected the now empty plastic bag Allan had brought into the emergency room from his car, and stuffed it into her pocket. Then she went back to work.

2

The inspection in the three-quarter mirror hanging behind the Rosewood credenza in his office was a ritual for Albert Averell Anthony, the administrator of Coit Hill Memorial Medical Center. And this morning, as usual, Anthony liked what he saw reflected there.

True, as far as he was concerned, he had not managed to erase all traces of his South Philadelphia Italian ancestry. He still thought of himself as somewhat too dark, looked with some distaste on the shape of his nose and, on occasion, cursed the too-black, too-thick texture of his hair. But the custom-tailored, three-piece silk suit (one of seven, the combined cost of which, he had recently calculated, could have financed a small Japanese automobile) was expertly cut to make him appear slimmer than he really was and even managed to give him an aura of understated elegance. The designer tie with its colorful, eye-catching pattern set against the expensive white-on-white shirt told the world that this was a man who, on occasion, liked to take chances.

With his left hand he brushed down his right shoulder and, after he had given his already perfectly knotted tie another tuck and had lifted it another half inch out of the vest so that the tie would not appear glued to his shirt, he decided he was ready. The day was one for which he had been preparing since the moment, almost fourteen months earlier, he had won the top job at Coit Hill Memorial Medical Center. In ten minutes he was scheduled to have breakfast with Richard "Rick" Marden, a banker and one of the most, if not the most, powerful member of Coit Hill Memorial's board of directors. At 10:30, the daily schedule on his desk noted, he was due to meet with Harvey Wallace, one of Coit Hill's key anesthesiologists. And at 12:30 he had an appointment with Sherman Harper, the head of the hospital's restructured cardiology department, grandly named the Coit Hill Memorial Heart Institute. For the briefest of moments, as he ran his finger down his calendar, Anthony wondered whether he should not have provided for some way to avoid the meetings with the anesthesiologist and cardiologist in case his meeting with Marden did not work out as anticipated. But he banished the idea almost as soon as it occurred to him. Marden would listen to him and give him the leeway to do exactly what he wanted.

Anthony strode purposefully through the heavy oak door into the reception area where his executive secretary and another personal secretary were already laboring. One was busy organizing her own day, while the other woman had started in on the stack of letters he had dictated the night before. Much like other missives he issued almost daily, these were letters addressed to other hospital administrators in the county, to county officials, to the hospital's board of directors, to prominent San Francisco citizens, to letters editors on local newspapers. The letters were worded differently, they even dealt with different subjects. But the common thread running through all of them was the message Anthony wanted to impart to the people who mattered in San Francisco: that Coit Hill Memorial was a medical institution determined to make its mark, one that was striving mightily to be the most prestigious hospital in the Bay area. With a cheery, "Good morning, girls," he strode past the women and out the glass double doors.

As he walked to the executive dining room where he was scheduled to meet with Marden, he tried but couldn't ignore the paper-strewn nursing stations, the feeding carts already brimming with empty breakfast dishes, the spots on the floors, the dirty ashtrays. To a man who kept the top of his desk clean of everything but his calendar, a leather-bound blotter, and a telephone, the clutter and mess were galling. On this day especially they were just one more reminder that though within a year he had managed to save Coit Hill Memorial from bankruptcy, there was still a long way to go before the hospital could live up to the vision he had for it. In another six months, he said to himself as he pushed open the doors of the dining room, there wouldn't be a Band-Aid out of place.

Marden was already sitting at a small table at the far side of the room, a cup of coffee in front of him cooling as he read the front page of the San Francisco *Telegraph*. As he always did when he met with Marden, Anthony wondered why he did not bother to get himself a good toupee. With a full set of hair to set off his dark eyes, aquiline nose, and square jaw, Marden, Anthony was sure, would be a good-looking man.

Anthony waved to Marden, then walked to the buffet to load a tray with toast, cereal, orange juice, and a coffeepot. After he had given Marden a hearty handshake he settled down to eat.

"So," Marden finally said after they had spent ten minutes of halfhearted chatter on the dismal showing the Giants were making so early in the new baseball season, "What's on the agenda for this morning?"

Despite the months he had spent planning the moves he was about to propose, despite the hours he had dedicated to learning the details of the speech he was about to deliver, Anthony felt his heart skip a beat or two. He had battled to pay and study his way first through an undergraduate degree at Temple University, then through two postgraduate degrees at the University of Michigan School of Public Health. In the ten years since he had left Ann Arbor he had jumped from hospital job to hospital job, simultaneously working his way up the executive ladder. The administrator's job he had landed at Coit Hill Memorial represented the culmination of a dream. If he offended Marden with the ideas he was about to present, he would be writing his resignation letter within a matter of months and would be forced to look elsewhere once again. But the doubts passed almost as quickly as they had come. He launched his assault.

"We've come a long way in the last few months to stabilize Coit financially," Anthony said. "But it's time to move on. We can't keep on running the hospital on a hand-to-mouth basis."

"We haven't done all that badly," Marden said, in a noncommittal tone. "True, we may not be as prestigious a hospital in the Bay area as you seem to think we should be, but we do our share. We serve the community around us, we do well by our patients."

"That's all true, but that sort of thing isn't good enough anymore," Anthony said, pouring more coffee for both of them. "Look, I'll give you an example. Almost forty percent of our beds right now are taken by patients who depend in one way or another on either the federal or the state government to pay their bills. We're losing money on every one of those patients."

"And what do you propose to do that would be better?" Marden asked.

Anthony didn't answer immediately. Marden, a man known for his temper and strong emotions, was also highly considered in San Francisco for his dedication to charities and service organizations that worked with the poor. When Anthony first came to Coit he'd tried to learn as much as possible about the influential people with whom he would be working; thus he knew that Marden's efforts in behalf of the downtrodden had their roots in deeply felt social commitment. Marden was well off and his family had been wealthy for at least two generations. Marden really felt that the haves should help the have-nots.

Anthony put down his cup of coffee and locked his eyes with Marden's. "We have to do away with as much of our poor population as possible and—"

"I beg your pardon?"

"I know it sounds hard, but there is no other way to put it. We have to diminish the number of uninsured people we accept at the hospital. We have too many illegal aliens, too many unemployed. They bring in nothing. They usually have a lot of problems, need a lot of care, use up a lot of services, and take up a lot of our bed space. What we need to do is get more and more patients who pay one hundred percent of their way."

"I don't think I have to remind you that we built at least two wings of Coit Hill Memorial with federal funds that came with a very strong string attached requiring us to provide care to people who had no other means of buying medical services. Or do I?"

"I am well aware of that. But right now we are caring for about seventy-five percent more poverty-level people than we have to in order to fulfill our obligations under the Hill-Burton law."

"And exactly what is to become of those people?" Anthony couldn't be absolutely sure, but sensed that Marden's voice had not carried the cold note that would have shown that he disapproved completely of his ideas.

"I'm not saying they shouldn't get care. Hell, give them to the county hospital, give them to S.F.U. Med Center. They can take care of them, probably better than we can."

Marden took his turn pouring coffee for the two of them. "I take it that is not the full extent of your plan to put Coit Hill Memorial in the black?"

"No, sir," Anthony said with a laugh. "It gets worse. We also have to start cutting down on the percentage of retired people who are covered under government plans. To be blunt about it, too many of them come to the hospital just to die. And since neither California nor the Feds cover the full cost of their care, it costs us an awful lot to house these people until they either go into a convalescent hospital or finally die. And with every level of government cutting back more and more on what they are willing to pay for, things are going to get even worse, believe me."

For the first time Marden looked at Anthony with something approaching distaste. "You're quite the humanitarian, aren't you?"

"It has nothing to do with humanitarianism, it has to do with running a hospital that won't go broke in another year. Look, if it'll make you feel better, I'd vote for any politician who is in favor of a national health insurance program and not just because it would maybe make us a few dollars. But that is not relevant right now. Hospitals are not charitable institutions, they are businesses. They have to make money to stay in business to render services to their customers. If you and the other directors want to, go on having the hospital do charity work. But in a year there won't be a Coit Hill Memorial left to help anyone, let alone the poor and the old."

"And where do you propose we get the people to fill the beds all those people will leave empty?"

"Piece of cake," Anthony said. "Give me a list of all the corporation presidents your bank does business with or that you and the other board members know personally. We'll offer them and their executives special programs for checkups, weight reduction, physical conditioning, whatever they need or want. Some of them will already have personal physicians, but most won't. When they go for their checkups, we put them in touch with docs who have privileges at Coit. In a year we will have built up a strong clientele among the executives and the docs, a clientele that is very grateful to us."

"Maybe. But even if it works, that won't be enough to fill beds."

Anthony saw he had Marden fully involved in listening to him. He decided to unveil the next part of his plan. "You know that eight-story building next to the hospital?"

"Yes, I know it. Eight or ten physicians who were on the staff here put together a syndicate to construct it. As a matter of fact, they arranged their financing through my bank."

"And have you kept track of how they are doing?"

"No. There hasn't been any reason to. They've been meeting their payments."

"They have, but not because the building has been making money. The building never reached full occupancy, so the partners in the syndicate have had to shell out money to make up the difference between what the building generates in rent and the amount of the mortgage with your bank."

"Why hasn't there been sufficient demand for the space?"

"How many doctors in San Francisco are busting their behinds to have staff privileges at Coit Hill Memorial and place their patients with us? And, aside from the convenience of being next to our hospital, why would anyone rent space in the building next to it?"

"Are you saying that they are close to defaulting?"

"I'm saying they are having trouble and, just between the two of us, they are going to have further trouble. Two of the doctors in the syndicate just can't afford another hike in their assessments for the mortgage. I would say the syndicate is in a position where it might soon default on the loan. And I would say they would be willing to listen to a reasonable offer for the building. What I'm suggesting is that the hospital offer to bail them out, to assume the loan, even pay them some of their equity."

"You think the hospital will have better luck drawing tenants and making the building viable?"

"You bet! For us the building won't be an investment so that we can all send our children to college. It'll be a tool to help us rebuild the hospital. We'll draw doctors by giving them a break on their rent, say a year's rent free or some kind of subsidy, whatever is necessary to get them to move in. We'll make our labs and diagnostic facilities available to them at a discount, maybe even pay for their membership in the terrific health spa we'll put into the new building. While the doctors are getting their day's portion of fitness, we'll have their cars washed. Or we'll convert this dining room into a private dining room just for physicians and provide gourmet meals."

"You know, Al, at one time or another we have considered some of your other ideas. They are not all that original."

"I never claimed they were original. Show me a successful hospital in any city and I'll show you a hospital run by people who not only adopted old ideas but then improved on them. Coit Hill Memorial hasn't done it because until last year it didn't have the kind of administration or board of directors that wanted to bother with putting any of these things into execution."

"Maybe because some of us still think hospitals should be run for the benefit of the community. Maybe it was because no one saw any reason to stir things up."

"That I know. All you have to do is look around and see the way the doctors run the hospital to figure out why."

"You seriously believe that, Al—that the doctors run this hospital?"

"It's not an illusion, Rick. Shortly before I got here the

radiologists started to campaign for one of the third-generation CAT scanners. If they were to practice at this hospital and remain competitive, they said, they had to have it. Never mind that it would cost over three-quarters of a million dollars. Never mind that I could count on less than one hand the number of patients who would have benefitted more from a third-generation than a second-generation scanner. But by golly, the doctors wanted it, and they almost got it."

"As I recall you put a stop to that. My phone rang for days after you made that decision."

"Sure I put a stop to it. A good thing I got here before the final contract was signed. Too bad I wasn't in time for some other things."

"Like?"

"How many ophthalmologists have privileges with Coit Hill Memorial? Three? Four? Two years ago we spent close to a million dollars for their toys, some of which are of questionable value, the rest of which will benefit even fewer patients than a third-generation CAT scanner. Name any department and I can give you examples. And don't even get me started on the Buck Rogers equipment the orthopods ordered and got. Whatever some of these egotistical maniacs wanted, the previous administrator gave them. Because, as you put it, no one wanted to stir them up. Because it would have been too much trouble to say no."

"Seems to me, Al, that you don't like doctors very much. Doesn't seem like a very healthy attitude, so to speak."

"I guess when it comes right down to it, no, I don't like them. They're a bunch of self-centered bastards who think they are more important than they really are. Doctors don't have much to do with the dispensation of medical care. Hell, give me a dozen competent nurses, a dozen competent nurse-practitioners, and a couple of doctors who know that they are just fancy mechanics, and I'll give you a hospital that puts money in the bank."

"Well, okay," Marden said, lighting the third cigarette since he had finished his food. "But has it ever occurred to you that your predecessor gave those people their toys, as you put it, because he basically subscribed to your philosophy that in order to get patients into the hospital you have to keep doctors happy?"

"Well, if that's what he was trying to do, he was going about it the wrong way. Yes, you want to court doctors, but as a hospital you want to do it on your terms, not theirs. At the very least, if you go to all the trouble of keeping the docs happy, then at least you do it by giving them concessions that help bring in a lot of patients, not concessions that will lead them to hospitalize just one or two a week who have some esoteric disease process. And again, you have to bring in patients who are covered by private insurance, not some rinky-dink program being administered by a bureaucrat in Sacramento who'll knock down your bill by an automatic twenty percent and then take one hundred and eighty days to pay you."

Anthony stood and walked back to the buffet. As he scooped some scrambled eggs onto a fresh plate and framed the eggs with four strips of bacon, he could feel Marden contemplating him. He was sure the banker was wondering if perhaps the board had hired too ambitious an administrator, one who would cause more turmoil than any of them were willing to put up with.

"There's something else," Anthony said as he sat back down and draped his napkin across his knee.

"You're throwing out minorities and the elderly; you're going to find us executives to put in our beds; you're going to take over a building and turn it into a spa; and there's more?"

Anthony swallowed a mouthful of eggs. "Oh, all of that will help. Everything else being equal we could have this institution completely turned around, maybe even showing a small profit within another twelve or eighteen months."

"I would say that in itself would be quite an accomplishment."

"It would be an accomplishment, but it wouldn't be enough. Delivery of health care is changing, Rick. Any hospital that wants to survive into the next decade is going to have to do more than just find new ways to cut corners or find new ways to do more gall bladders."

Marden's face showed he was not sure where Anthony was leading, but the banker made no move to interject a comment or ask a question. "I think we should look for ways to make Coit Hill more than just a hospital," Anthony continued. "What we should do is look to turn it into a real medical center, into an institution that will hold its own against the most prestigious hospitals in this area."

Marden still said nothing. Anthony paused, wondering if the silence signaled the banker's way of giving him leeway to calculate how far he could go.

"I think we can start working on that too," Anthony went on, though with some hesitation. "What I'd like to do is institute a new service that will bring us a lot of publicity, put Coit Hill in everyone's mind, whether they use us or not, and, of course, generate a good deal of income."

"And the way to do that is?"

"Put in a trauma service."

"A trauma service?" Marden questioned. "Now look . . ."

"I know what you're going to say," Anthony answered. "More emergency-room physicians and surgeons the hospital will have to pay. Too expensive."

"Precisely. On top of subsidizing the building next door, I'd say all that is too much, even if you achieve all the cost savings you're talking about. I think a trauma service is something we can put on the back burner for a while." Marden took the napkin off his lap, folded it, and put it on the table. He started to push his chair away from the table.

"Rick," Anthony said, almost too abruptly. "Trust me with this. We can crank up enough of a trauma service to get some visibility in the community without spending millions. And besides . . . ," Anthony stopped and smiled broadly, "I have just the way to finance the trauma service and our costs on the building next door. It won't cost the hospital a penny."

Marden drained the last few drops of coffee and looked at his watch. "I'd love to hear the details, but I've got another meeting. I'm leaving town in a couple of days for about three weeks. Let's talk again when I get back."

Anthony's right hand balled into a fist. "I hate to press you, but there are a couple of decisions coming up before then that could influence whether or not we can put in a trauma service in the next year."

Marden stood, then pushed his chair back toward the table. "All right, Al. Draw up a memo on your financing ideas and get it to my office before I leave. If you want to take some preliminary steps, go ahead. But make damned sure you don't overextend yourself . . . or us."

As he walked back to his office, Anthony could barely contain his glee. He had always thought that Marden, like most lay professionals, held doctors in especially high esteem, and his suspicion had been confirmed by the expression on the other man's face when Anthony had criticized the hospital's previous administration for catering to doctors' demands for new high-tech equipment. Anthony suspected that Marden would be distressed when he learned that the purchase of the medical building and the financing of the trauma center hinged on a financial campaign Anthony had, in fact, already launched against a selected few of the specialists on the hospital staff. But he also was convinced that Marden would do nothing to stop his plans.

Six months earlier Anthony had summoned a cardiologist and a neurologist to his office for separate meetings. Both were partners in the syndicate that owned the building next door to the hospital. Both had lucrative contracts with Coit Hill under which each man received $100,000 a year to provide consulting services to already hospitalized patients—the cardiologist to read and interpret EKGs, the neurologist to run the neurodiagnostic laboratory. Pleading the hospital's strained financial condition, Anthony had cut their contract in half. The doctors had protested, but did not fight the decision, confirming Anthony's suspicion that he had considerable latitude for maneuvering. Just as important, the cutback in their income forced both men to pull out as part owners of the building Anthony coveted. Between the time Anthony had cut the contracts and the week preceding that morning's meeting with Marden, the syndicate had not been able to find two other investors to replace the two doctors. Word indeed was out that the building would soon be for sale. As he entered his office, Anthony reminded himself to call the hospital's attorney that afternoon to have him begin the process of buying out the syndicate.

The next physician Anthony had targeted, Harvey Wallace, the hospital's leading anesthesiologist, was now idly leafing through a leisure magazine in the reception area while waiting for Anthony. The administrator ushered him into the office, offered him a seat, then moved briskly to his side of the desk and sat down. While Wallace sat staring at him, Anthony studied a massive computer printout he had taken out of the top drawer of the desk. Anthony made an elaborate show of running his index finger down column after column of figures. But he knew by heart the statistics he was about to use against Wallace. Finally he put aside the sheaf of papers and looked up at Wallace.

"As close as I can make out, Dr. Wallace, you and the eleven other anesthesiologists who are on staff here billed patients for close to four-point-four million dollars last year, is that right?"

Wallace, taken aback by the direct reference to finances, was immediately alarmed. "Well, I don't know about—"

"Four million, four hundred and sixty thousand dollars, to be exact, doctor," Anthony snapped back before lapsing into a dead silence and looking directly and intently at Wallace.

Wallace had heard talk about the EEG and EKG contract, but had paid scant attention to the murmurs of nervousness among some of his colleagues. He didn't know the physicians involved very well and, besides, he had always thought the contracts the cardiologists and neurologists had with the hospital were boondoggles. Half of the tests those men interpreted should probably never have been ordered in the first place. The other half could be read by competent residents at a fraction of the money the hospital had so willingly paid for years. Wallace had never contemplated the possibility that Anthony would turn his attention to the anesthesiologists. Their work, after all, was absolutely necessary. "But, that's . . . well, I mean, twelve anesthesiologists . . . ," he stammered, not knowing immediately what to say.

"It's too much, Dr. Wallace," Anthony said. "At least from the point of view of this institution. I can't let that continue."

"I'm sorry, I don't think I understood. What do you mean you can't let it continue?"

Anthony made a conscious effort to harden his face. "From now on, doctor, anesthesiology at this hospital will be performed on a contractual basis. Roughly speaking, the terms of the contract are these: The man heading the anesthesiology department will be paid an annual fee of two hundred thousand dollars and he will be renewed on a year-to-year basis. Among his other duties, he will hire the other anesthesiologists who will work at the hospital. I would guess that he would be offering them year-to-year contracts and pay them about seventy-five to eighty-five thousand dollars a year."

"And you'll cut the charges to the patients accordingly? You're quite mad, Anthony. Your fellow administrators at other hospitals around the Bay area will run you out of town."

"I never said I would cut what the patient is charged, Dr. Wallace. We'll still bill patients at the old rates. But the difference will go to the hospital."

"So what you are proposing to do is simply to appropriate about . . . ," Wallace stopped to carry out the mental calculations, then continued, "about three-point-two million dollars of our money. You think you can get away with it?"

Anthony reached for a manila folder and, using the same deliberate air he had devoted to the computer printout, scrutinized the folder's contents. "Let's see now, correct me if I'm wrong. You're divorced and have two kids by that marriage. The boy is at Harvard, second year medical student. The girl is tucked away at a finishing school in Missouri. You're still making payments on the house your ex-wife lives in with that sensitive poet she threw you over for—"

"Now see here, Anthony . . ."

"Wait, wait. Let's go on. You're married now to a twenty-eight-year-old lawyer who works for the public defender's office. What's she making, twenty thou a year? The two of you have a three-year-old kid who has a full-time nanny, a real English one who isn't working for peanuts, while Mommy and Daddy are off at work."

"All right, Anthony, I know the details of my financial life." Wallace's voice was rising, as was the color in his face. "What's the point?"

"The point is that you could use the two hundred thousand

dollars a year we'd pay the head of the group. Play ball with me and assume the job as head of anesthesia, hire the other people, and everyone lives happily ever after."

The two men stared at each other, smug self-satisfaction in Anthony's eyes, loathing in Wallace's. "So in a way I have to do your dirty work for you," Wallace finally said, "and go out and tell my colleagues that they will have to take a massive cut in compensation if they want to go on working here. And if they refuse?"

"If they refuse? Let me read you the one hundred and thirty enquiries this hospital has had in the last twelve months from anesthesiologists who are tired of fighting Chicago's winters, Detroit's depression economy, and New York's muggings, and who would give up their last drop of Pentothal to come to San Francisco. And when we're through with those we can go through all the applications from graduates of a couple of medical schools in the Caribbean who are looking for starting positions as resident anesthesiologists. We'd fill any open positions in forty-eight hours, doctor."

Wallace got up and walked to the door. "I'll think about it and let you know." Anthony, wanting to leave the man a little bit of his dignity, refrained from pointing out that he had already made up his mind. Feeling immensely pleased with himself, Anthony buzzed his executive secretary and asked her to take some dictation before his scheduled lunch with Sherman Harper, his star cardiac surgeon.

Harper had been one of Anthony's first triumphs after taking over as administrator at Coit Hill. At the time Sherman Harper had been at the San Francisco University Medical Center. The tall, graying man whose angular face was dominated by bulging eyes was one of the city's most distinguished cardiac surgeons. His reputation went far beyond San Francisco's city limits. But Sherman Harper had not been a happy man. He had come to San Francisco from Baylor University, lured not only by the prospect of living in a city he had long loved from afar, but by the promises the University had made: an opportunity for him to build a strong cardiac surgery residency, the chance to design and build his very own operating rooms and intensive-care unit, a chance to run whatever research programs he needed to advance his already considerable knowledge of lipid metabolism and its role in the onset of coronary artery disease.

The promises had been well intentioned and honest. But most of them had not come about, largely because the University, facing tremendous budgetary cutbacks as a result of the state government's effort to prune back its own expenditures, could no longer afford to go ahead with the bright promises it had waved before Harper's eyes. And Harper had begun to put out feelers for a new position.

Anthony had heard of Harper's dissatisfaction when a friend in the administrative offices of the University of Michigan's Medical Center mentioned in a casual, touching-base telephone conversation that Harper had been looking seriously at an offer to come to Ann Arbor. Within minutes after hanging up the phone, Anthony had called a special meeting of the board of directors' executive committee. After a good deal of debate (much of it heated), the committee bought Anthony's proposals that a goodly portion of the $4.5 million that had been put aside toward making the hospital more earthquake-resistant be invested in building the city's finest cardiac care unit. A few days later Anthony had called Harper and had arranged to meet with him. There would be no pussyfooting around, Anthony had decided. He would hit Harper with his offer head on.

During that meeting almost ten months earlier, Anthony had outlined his offer, one that would give Harper the chance to do much of what the University had not allowed him to accomplish.

The cardiac surgeon had listened patiently to Anthony's speech. "You have to understand, Anthony, that I moved out here on the basis of promises that were not kept," Harper had said when Anthony finally stopped. "And while your interest is flattering, I am fully aware that your institution does not seem to have the financial resources to back up its offer."

Anthony had walked back to his desk and reached for an envelope lying on top of the otherwise bare surface. He rejoined Harper and, deliberately saying nothing, opened the envelope, took out a check, and placed it on the glass-and-chrome table in front of them. "That, Dr. Harper, is a check for two and three-quarters million dollars," Anthony had said at the time. "If you accept our offer, you and I will go down to the bank and open a special account. You'll be the only one authorized to draw on that account and, so long as you give me reports on your progress every three months or so, there'll be no questions asked. I know that is not enough to set up a complete heart institute, but it is more than enough to at least start a good one. In other words, there'll be more in time."

Harper went about spending the money with relish and abandon. He converted Coit Hill Memorial's fifth floor into the gleaming "Coit Hill Memorial Heart Institute." A new operating suite was busy virtually every day from 6:30 in the morning until late in the afternoon. The Institute's cardiac care unit contained all the latest electronic gadgetry. The cardiac rehabilitation program—oriented to people who had had bypass surgery or who had had heart attacks but did not want an operation—drew not only patients from Coit Hill but referrals from other hospitals as well. Executives who did not want to court heart attacks came to the Institute's Cardiac Conditioning classes, its stop-smoking workshops. They even brought their wives to the Institute's cooking classes where the women could learn to prepare meals virtually free of cholesterol and saturated fats. When not busy operating or seeing patients, Harper was working feverishly to put together his Institute's first symposium, a meeting that would bring heart specialists from all over the United States to Coit Hill Memorial for scientific exchanges or refresher courses. Anthony had succeeded in turning Harper into a happy man.

Striding back into the executive dining room at 12:35, Anthony could see, however, that on this particular day Harper was anything but pleased. Still brimming with satisfaction over his meetings with Marden and Wallace, Anthony chose to ignore the older man's very apparent gloom. He greeted Harper heartily, then turned to the balding young man also sitting at the table, Bernard Claudet, the hospital's general manager, an accounting genius Anthony had lured away from one of the city's leading accounting firms.

"How goes it, Bernie?" Anthony asked. "Did you bring the pro forma?"

"Yes, I have the figures." Claudet pushed a manila folder toward Anthony's seat.

Harper, his seething anger growing more obvious, bolted up from his seat. "If you'll excuse me," he said curtly, "I think I'll get something to eat."

Anthony threw an inquisitive look at Claudet, but the accountant merely shrugged. The administrator followed the surgeon to the buffet line.

Saying nothing, the two men picked up their trays, silverware, and napkins. Anthony chose a fruit salad, Harper a plate of steaming linguini with clams.

"Sherman, you look like you're going to have a coronary," Anthony said in a low voice as they stopped before the selection of small bottles of California wines and imported beers. "Want to get it off your chest?"

"If you are saying that I'm angry, you're damned right," Harper said as he snatched a bottle out of the crushed ice and slammed it onto his tray. "After working hard on cases all day and having to come down to resect an emergency aneurysm at midnight, I don't appreciate being woken up at three in the morning by some goddamn snotty E.R. doc who—"

"Hold on a minute," Anthony interrupted. "What the hell are you talking about?"

Harper picked an apple tart out of the display of desserts and slapped it on his tray. "At three this morning somebody named Kirk calls me from the E.R. room. He's got some kid who has been in a bike-car crunch. From what he tells me over the phone I know the kid is as good as dead. But no, he insists, I mean the son of a bitch practically ordered me to come down to operate. Who does—"

Anthony picked up his tray. "Did you turn down the case?" He asked as he led the way back to the table.

"I told you the son of a bitch practically ordered me down."

They reached the table where Claudet, who had gone through the line even before Harper had arrived, was already sipping his coffee.

"And you want to know why I am angry?" he said as they emptied their trays on the table. "Because this bastard not only has the gall to tell me that he'll hold me responsible if the kid dies without surgery, but then when I get in here—" Harper, well aware that the dining room was nearly full, bent toward Anthony and struggled to keep his temper from driving his voice into a shout, "—the kid is dead! Just as I said he would be."

Anthony tried to be conciliatory. "Look, I'm sorry, the guy shouldn't have bothered you."

"You're damned right he shouldn't have. Who the hell needs that kind of grief? With my schedule, I don't need middle-of-the-night calls on two-bit cases."

Anthony looked up from his salad. "I am afraid, though, Sherman, that you may have to accept those calls, at least for a while."

"Listen, I know that I'm also acting as chief of staff, but the understanding was clearly that it was to be a nominal designation. I repeat. I don't want the grief that goes with it."

"Sherman, I know you don't. But for a while you are going to have to put up with it. I want to start drawing more emergency cases here and I've worked out a deal that would get ambulances to bring us people from car wrecks, that sort of thing."

"A deal? What kind of a deal? With whom?"

Anthony laughed at the suspicious tone that had crept into Harper's voice. "About four years ago the Board of Supervisors cut the county into four so-called emergency zone areas. In each of them, one hospital has a two-way radio in its emergency room. It is supposed to use the radio first to help the paramedics on the scene of a problem assess the situation and start the right kind of treatment and second to direct the paramedics to the nearest hospital with the capability of handling the patient, either because it has an ICU bed free or some kind of specialized service. But in reality none of those hospitals ever direct a patient anywhere but into their own E.R. rooms."

"Let me guess," Harper said. "Now we are going to have a radio too."

"You're quick, doctor. In the last supervisorial election two of our board members put twenty-five thousand dollars into the campaign of the guy who heads the board's emergency care services subcommittee. It wasn't too hard to convince him that the county really did need one more base station. And we're it."

"Are you nuts?" Harper asked, staring at Anthony as if the man had suddenly announced that he wanted the doctors in the hospital to start using leeches again. "You want hippie accident victims dragged in here, or prostitutes whose pimps have put butcher knives up their cunts because they've been holding back some of the receipts? You want all the bums who in their stupor walk in front of cable cars? What the hell are you talking about?"

"I'm talking about cashing in on something we've been ignoring, something that will get us more patients for our beds and for some of the doctors who aren't as fortunate as you are. I'm talking about getting insurance bucks that are now going to other hospitals around here, including, you should pardon the expression, the University."

"Al, I'm asking you again. Are you nuts? Half the people who get banged up on the Bayshore or who get stabbed or shot in the Haight haven't got dime one. So where the hell are you going to make money on them?"

"We're going to make money because we're not going to get a hell of a lot of the indigent cases you're worrying about. Most of those fall in the University's catchment area. We'll get a few poverty cases in here, sure. But so what? If we get someone with no insurance all we have to do is stabilize him, then transfer him to the county hospital. But when the paramedics bring in someone who has been in a wreck or has been shot and is covered by insurance, he stays here."

"So what you're saying is that we should come running in in the middle of the night, screw up our elective schedules and who knows what else just for the sake of operating on the dead and making a couple of bucks?"

"A lot more than a couple of bucks. If you had pulled the kid out and, say that he was insured, that would have meant fifty to a hundred grand, minimum, for the care he would have gotten. Multiply that by five hundred or so cases a year, and you'll see what we're talking about here. And some individual cases could mean as much as one million dollars in billings to insurance companies."

"Yeah, Al, I know what we're talking about. We're talking

about greed and delusions of grandeur. It's not worth it, Al."

"It's worth it because we are talking about more than the insurance money they'll bring in, and you know it, Sherman. As word gets around about our new Trauma Treatment Center—"

"Our what?"

"Our Trauma Treatment Center. As word gets around the Bay about that, other patients with other problems will start demanding to come here, even if they only have to have a hysterectomy, a nose job, or a prostate. They'll figure if we can bring people back from the dead, we'll be able to do other miracles for them. Give me five more years and this will be one of the top regional hospitals in the Bay area. And that'll rub off on you as well."

"You make it sound simple, Al. But you're forgetting something, aren't you? There aren't three surgeons on staff here who give a damn about trauma. I certainly don't. Who the hell wants to be on call to come and do those cases? Trauma cases will just overburden us and get in the way of everything else we're trying to do. Let those patients go to the University and let us stick to our business."

"Our business is to stay alive as an institution, Sherman. We can't do that unless we keep growing. Right now you and that Institute we've got sitting up there on the fifth floor are going great guns. But your biggest moneymakers right now are still the coronary bypasses you do. What's to guarantee that the bypass will remain as the treatment of choice for plugged arteries? Percutaneous transluminal angioplasty is coming up fast and it's a hell of a lot cheaper than bypass surgery. There are several people working on using laser beams to ream out clogged arteries. The Institute is doing well now, but you could be out of business in five years. Or, if the heart attack rate keeps dropping . . ."

"Pipe dreams, Al. Come on, leave the blue-skying to medical writers."

"Okay, maybe it's blue-skying. But the point is that I'm serious about building a trauma service that is a profit center, Sherman. We're going to go all out on this." Anthony turned to Claudet. "Did you bring the pro forma on the helicopter?"

"It's in the folder in front of you."

Anthony opened the folder and scanned the papers inside. "It'll work financially for us?"

"It'll work . . . if Marden's shipping friend comes through with the donation he's talking about. The chopper will cost us about half a million dollars. Building the helipad won't be that much, maybe a few grand to put a concrete landing zone out on the front lawn. But the upkeep, paying the pilots for twenty-four-hour duty, that sort of thing will cost us at least another half a million a year."

Looking at Harper, Anthony had to repress a laugh. The doctor's eyes were virtually out of their sockets. "A million dollars for a helicopter," the surgeon said. "A million dollars? We've got equipment in this hospital that's twenty-five years old, this building still doesn't meet earthquake codes and is going to come down around our ears in the next major quake, we need a dozen more nurses, and you want to spend a million dollars on a helicopter?"

"Sure, it'll do wonders for us."

"Al, the radiology department is still pissed because they didn't get their new CAT scanner. And now you're going to go out and spend a million on a helicopter. It makes no sense."

"Sure it makes sense. A CAT scanner is metallic gray, bulky, sits in our basement and is seen by two radiologists, one nurse, and a few scared-out-of-their-wits patients a week. A helicopter will be seen by hundreds of thousands of people a week who'll see it whiz by or who'll see it on the tube because every time we dispatch it we'll make sure the television news programs know about it. Beyond its medical uses that chopper will tell people we're dynamic, active, involved."

"What kind of medical uses are you talking about, for God's sake? You've got the base station, you just said that it will help you draw from the pool of trauma victims. This is San Francisco, Anthony, not Los Angeles County. A helicopter is practically out of the county's limits before it takes off."

"Why worry just about patients who are within the San Francisco limits? Why shouldn't we have a shot at trauma patients in Marin County, or in Contra Costa County?"

"You're mad, Al, you really are. I can just see what's going to happen. The base station is going to pick up a call on a badly injured patient two miles from here, and while the paramedics are trying to get there in their ambulance your bird is going to swoop down from the skies and pluck the patient off for Coit Hill Memorial. And when you hear about somebody wrapped around a telephone pole over in San Rafael, off goes the helicopter and kidnaps the patient and flies him all the way back here. All for your glory?"

"Not my glory, Sherman. For the patient's good. The faster the patient gets care, the better off he is. You know that Sherman, even if you don't know much about trauma."

"I know enough to know that if I were the patient, I sure as hell wouldn't want a paramedic struggling to stabilize me in a cramped, bucking and flopping helicopter when he could just as well be doing it comfortably and a hell of a lot safer in a roomy ambulance. I could see it if we were the only competent trauma service within one hundred miles and if we had to bring in patients from the boonies somewhere. But this is unnecessary grandstanding, Al. I won't be a part of it."

"It's not grandstanding at all, Sherman. And Sherman, you'll be a part of it."

"You can certainly get your center set up without involving me," Harper said, returning to his linguini as if the conversation was over and the point settled.

"I want this," Anthony persisted, refusing to let the doctor dismiss him, "and you're going to help me. You owe me, Sherman. I don't like to remind you of that, but you do. And you're going to help me. I gave you a chance to revive your career and do things you couldn't have done anywhere else."

"And just what do you expect me to do?"

"Serve as interim head of the Trauma Center. Organize it. Go out into the community and talk it up at all those Lion and Elk and other funny animal clubs that invite you to talk about the heart-disease epidemic while they wolf down their high-cholesterol lunches."

"I'm a cardiac surgeon, Al," Sherman Harper said, a hint of a whine creeping into his voice, the whine of a child who knows he is fighting a losing battle. "I haven't done trauma since Korea and I was damned glad when I did my last case then. Not to mention that trauma care has gone through a revolution even since Vietnam. I am way out of touch, Al."

"Learn, Sherman." The hard edge was back in Anthony's voice. Harper looked away and Anthony knew he had won. In victory he was generous. "Give it a year, Sherman. Do you know Everett Huntington at the University?"

Harper shook his head.

"He's an E.R. physician," Anthony went on. "Has been there since just after the Vietnam war. Without going into details, he's another one the University has screwed over. Hire him away, Sherman, and make him director of our E.R. at a hundred thou or something like that and guarantee him a life free from political problems. Once you get him, he can build the E.R. and you can pull back from that."

"And the surgical support?"

"Hire that too, Sherman. We've got the dough for it." Anthony stopped and regarded the surgeon. "Sherman, don't sulk."

"I wasn't aware that I was sulking."

"All I'm really asking is for you to loan your name and some of your organizational skills to this project. Once we've got it started you'll be out of it and you'll have all the time you need to mess around in your lipid metabolism lab."

Harper cringed, catching a faintly amused look from Claudet, who had been silently observing the entire exchange. A searing hatred for Anthony and his manipulations surged through the doctor. "So what you're telling me," he said finally, "is that if I'm a good little boy and do your bidding, you'll finally get around to authorizing the construction of that lab. Is that right?"

"I don't care what kind of an interpretation you put on things, Sherman, just so you recall what you owe this institution."

3

The grating sound of the foghorn cut through the still night, its deep, sorrowful tone carrying into Allan's bedroom.

To Allan, who at two in the morning was still wide awake and staring at the ceiling, it was a petulant voice, punctuating the uneasy feelings that had been plaguing him since the biker had died at Coit Hill Memorial a week earlier. How was it possible that a hospital accepting trauma cases could have a call list made up of surgeons who could not be found when they were needed and of vacationing surgeons who asked physicians without privileges at Coit Hill Memorial to cover for them? How could the hospital's administration appoint physicians to trauma if those specialists could simply refuse to come in? But a more basic question was also eating at Allan. Had he, in fact, been trying to save a patient who was already essentially dead? Perhaps the biker's injuries had been worse than he had thought; perhaps nothing, not even the most heroic of medical efforts, would have saved him. Yet Allan and his colleagues, in the more than three years during which he had been a part of the trauma team at the University Medical Center, had been able to save dozens of patients. Were those people who would have survived anyway, even in the worst of the community hospital emergency rooms?

He threw back the covers, got out of bed and walked to the window. There was little to see but the dense white fog and the dim streetlight below. He grabbed an old robe to throw over his naked body and shuffled off to the kitchen. The Swiss cuckoo clock perched above the breakfast table struck the quarter after the hour as he walked in. Can I have a beer? he asked himself. He decided he could. There were already two surgeons, David Fedder and Joe Santorre, on duty that night at the University. That meant he wouldn't be called in and didn't have to keep a clear head. With gusto he pulled open the refrigerator door, reached in and took a bottle of beer out of the six-pack he kept in there for the rare occasions when he allowed himself to savor a drink.

He eased himself into a chair, took a long swig, put the bottle down, and leaned back until the chair's two front legs were off the ground. He stared at the bottle intently, almost as if he expected a genie to rise from it and give him answers to the questions that had been careening through his brain. But the only thing the bottle seemed ready to supply him with were more questions. Maybe the biker's death was an exception, a fluke, maybe nothing could have saved him. Still, why did Allan keep hearing reports about seemingly unnecessary deaths from other residents who moonlighted at other hospitals around the county? If Coit Hill Memorial and the other institutions were staffing their E.R.'s with people who knew their business, why, at least three or four times a week, did ambulances come to the University Medical Center bearing half-dead patients who had first been admitted, then discharged from other emergency rooms?

There was no doubt, he decided. The evidence, though circumstantial, was telling him that a fair number of people were dying in emergency rooms not because their injuries were overwhelming—but because the hospitals to which they were taken just were not up to coping with their injuries. Allan allowed the chair to fall forward so that he could reach the bottle of beer. What he needed to do, his instincts told him, was find definitive proof that people were dying unnecessarily in E.R. rooms. Easily said, Allan, he chided himself. But how to do it?

And then the bottle of beer delivered up its genie.

On a Saturday about six months earlier, a wino had been

brought into the University emergency room after having been found near a ramp leading to the Bayshore Freeway. Within a few minutes of his admission to the emergency room he had suffered a heart attack and, despite desperate attempts to save him, had died. The man was well into his sixties and the paramedics, trying to keep up with the pace of a typically busy weekend night, had rushed away without giving David Fedder, who had been on duty at the time, any details about the wino's blood pressure. Later, Fedder, in signing the death certificate had simply listed "cardiac arrest" as the cause of death and had let it go at that.

A week later, Fedder, looking as if he had just been the object of an embarrassing lecture, had lumbered into the lounge reserved for residents.

"What's the matter with you?" Allan had asked at the time.

"Last week I was on when the paramedics brought in a wino they found on the Bayshore who then arrested on us. I just got a call from the medical examiner's office. The arrest was not the cause of death, not technically."

"It was secondary to shock?"

"Yeah. The post showed that his liver had been pulverized. Not to mention the fact that the iliac artery had ruptured. We wouldn't have saved his ass anyway, but he arrested because he lost blood, not because of a myocardial infarction or underlying heart disease."

"Okay, terrific. But why'd they do a post on the guy? It wasn't exactly a suspicious death."

"Didn't have to be just suspicious," Fedder answered. "The woman who called said that by law the M.E.'s office has to do an autopsy in every case where the mechanism of death is in doubt. Since he might have been in an accident, they just automatically presumed that we'd fucked up by putting down cardiac arrest as the event that caused the death and that it had been secondary to some other event. Well, they were right."

Suddenly, Allan leapt up from his chair, scurried to his bedroom, and rifled through the papers cluttering the top of his rolltop desk until he found the small address book in which he kept names and numbers of people with whom he had—or might someday have—professional contact. When Fedder had told the story, Allan asked him for the name of the woman from the medical examiner's office. Someone that conscientious might well be a good contact someday.

"Julie," he muttered to himself. "Julie what?" He flipped through each alphabetical listing until he came upon the name: Julie McDonough.

When he woke up, he was first upset because he had obviously slept through the alarm; then he realized he felt refreshed: even with the bout of insomnia, this was the first night in weeks in which he had had more than three or four hours of sleep. He called the hospital, arranged for someone to cover for him for the rest of the day, showered leisurely, shaved, dressed, and drove off to find Julie McDonough.

A few minutes after eleven he arrived at the medical examiner's office. The black woman at the reception desk eyed him coolly when he asked for Julie McDonough, then paged her on a public address system, the name reverberating through the long, empty halls leading away from the reception area.

Allan sat down in one of the lobby chairs to wait. Seated across from him was a young woman in old jeans and a faded tank top. Long, stringy blonde hair fell to her shoulders. A tattoo of a butterfly adorned the top of her left breast. As she absentmindedly stroked the head of a young girl sitting next to her, she stared out into space. He wondered idly who had died. A girl friend from an overdose? A boyfriend in a barroom brawl? A parent she had not paid attention to for ten years? Suddenly her gaze shifted and her eyes, full of grief, met Allan's. Taken aback, he looked away.

He took refuge in an old *Life* magazine, idly flipping through the pages, well aware that he had no idea what he would say to Julie McDonough. Though he knew what he wanted to find out, he didn't know how to go about it.

If he had any hopes of at least partially sorting out his thoughts, they were quickly shattered when he saw the woman coming toward him. Her legs, shaped by the high heels she was wearing, were long and strong. Though she was trim, her hips were ample and fluid. Above her narrow waist, her breasts bobbed softly against a simple silk blouse. Her face, open and expectant, was devoid of makeup. Her lips, full and outlined by a natural rose tint, were partly open in a smile. There were freckles across the bridge of her nose, and high cheekbones defined large, green eyes. Her cheeks radiated a warm, healthy glow. Thick, rust-colored hair cascaded below her shoulders. She looked about twenty-five years old.

The young woman stopped at the reception desk, then turned when the receptionist nodded toward Allan. "I'm Julie McDonough," she said while walking toward him and extending her hand.

Allan, his heart beating as if he had just finished the Boston Marathon, introduced himself as well as he could, then stopped.

"Glad to meet you, Dr. Kirk." There was a touch of laughter in her eyes as she waited for him to go on.

Embarrassed at his sudden inability to be coherent, Allan felt his cheeks grow warm. "Well," she said lightly, "there's a room over there we can use." She led him to a door a few steps down one of the hallways and showed him into a small room. One of the walls was glass, with a curtain drawn across its face. A small intercom was on a thin strip of wall immediately to the left of the window. An open box of paper tissues stood next to a lamp on the single table.

"Our viewing room for relatives," she explained. She sat down in one of the chairs next to the table and, with a movement of her hand, invited him to take the other seat. "What can I do for you, Dr. Kirk?"

"Allan is okay," he blurted.

She nodded. "Julie, then."

He took a deep breath and plunged ahead. "About six months ago you called one of our residents at the University hospital to tell him that a patient of ours had died not as a result of a cardiac arrest but from massive internal injuries he suffered in an accident."

Julie shrugged her shoulders. "I don't remember the case specifically, but if you are here to dispute the interpretation of the autopsy result, I'm not the one to—"

"No, no," he interrupted hurriedly. "No, that's not it. I was interested in why you called."

"I try to get around to every hospital and let them know when a finding here does not substantiate the cause of death as listed on the death certificate at the hospital."

"Do you keep a list of all the cases that come through here? I mean like a statistical compilation of real causes of death?"

"In part, yes. That's my job. I keep the statistics that tell us how many people have been murdered, how many suicides we have, that kind of thing. I'm the statistician here."

"How about statistics on deaths due to car accidents, industrial accidents, the like. Do you keep track of those?"

"We keep numbers on industrial stuff. We feed those routinely to government agencies interested in worker safety and to the Centers for Disease Control."

Allan allowed himself to get excited now. If they knew how many people died as a result of accidents and if the medical examiner's office called hospitals to let them know about causes of death as a result of accidents like the one the drunk had been involved in, Julie would be able to tell him exactly how many people died in accidents as a result of uncontrolled, internal bleeding. That might give him some indication of how many people were dying as a result of inadequate care at the various hospitals around the county.

His hopes, though, were quickly dashed. No, she told him, they kept track of how many people died in accidents, but not specifically of the mechanism of death in each case. "Officially, no one really cares," she said, "if someone died of a ruptured aorta or a transsected liver. The things most government agencies are interested in are suicide rates, murder rates, deaths from accidental poisonings, or accidents at home or on the job. So that's all we report. I call hospitals, as I called yours, and tell them the cause of death; but I don't bother keeping separate statistical records on that sort of thing. We have enough to do around here as it is."

Allan chewed on the inside of his lip, trying to think.

"Listen," she said after he had allowed a few seconds to lapse in silence. "Wouldn't it be much easier if you told me what you were looking for? I was about to go to lunch, if you want to join me. There's a good Mexican deli around the corner."

"Sure," Allan shot back, too enthusiastically, he was sure. "Thanks for asking."

"I'll get some money," she said. He watched her walk away, entranced by the sight of the wavy hair falling down her back, her straight, assured carriage, her round buttocks.

The "deli" was a very small, intensely crowded lunchroom. Allan counted a dozen people eating at the counter and almost as many people standing behind them waiting for stools. The floor area was crowded with cheap Salvation Army tables and chairs. Two fat waitresses were, in virtual nonstop motion, rushing in and out of a small door, in one trip carrying away dirty dishes, in the next trip bringing out plates overflowing with tamales, burritos, refried beans. A table opened up and Julie led Allan to it. They stood and waited as a busboy made a halfhearted attempt to wipe away the few crumbs and many spots the previous occupants had left behind.

Anticipating a long shift ahead of him at the hospital, Allan ordered a soft drink. Julie ordered a Dos Equis. The busboy scurried over with a basket of tortilla chips and two containers of hot sauce. Allan reached for the largest tortilla chip he could find and dipped it first into the bowl containing a red sauce, then into a bowl holding a greenish sauce with tiny specks floating around in it. He bit into the chip, shuddering as the full impact of the hot pepper sauces struck him. When he recovered his breath, he told her about the biker's death.

"Damned near wiped me out," he finished. "Obviously, we see a lot of people die all the time. But, Christ, the way this happened. Young, strapping kid, his whole life ahead of him—and I have to watch him bleed out because I can't get consultants in." He paused for another sauce-laden chip and followed it quickly with a sip of his drink. "Then I started to think. Another resident on the staff moonlighting at St. Xavier was telling us a while back about a woman who had been brought in to that E.R. one night he was on duty. She'd been wiped out in a crosswalk by a hit-and-run driver. Tried like hell to save her. Our guy called a surgeon and he said he'd be right there. And, relatively speaking, he was. He lived about forty-five minutes from the hospital and got there in thirty-five. She died ten minutes later while the surgeon was still scrubbing."

Julie said nothing. Her frank way of looking at him was still making him uncomfortable. "Not too long ago we get a call at the University from an E.R. doc at another hospital," he said. "Gas station attendant, some Iranian kid, gets shot in the stomach during a holdup at four in the morning. Medics get him into the hospital all right. He's bleeding like a pig, but there's a general surgeon in house. Had had a fight with his wife and was sleeping in an empty room. All the time in the world to pull the patient through, right? Guess what. No one can find the key to the operating room. Guy bleeds out in the E.R.

"Last month we hear of another case through the grapevine. Kid badly hurt when he falls off a cliff near a hiking trail. They bring him in to Cedars. The E.R. over there is terrific, I mean they bring cadavers back to life. Everyone works their butts off. But the E.R. can't get a surgeon in because it's five-thirty in the afternoon and no one within beeper distance can cut through the rush-hour traffic to get to the hospital in time."

He stopped as their waitress skidded up to their table. She threw his Machaca burrito in front of him, dumped Julie's carnitas in front of her, turned on her heels, and sped away. She must have known Julie as a regular because in seconds she was back with another bottle of beer.

"What I want to know—" the thought finally working its way out of Allan's subconscious—"is whether those were flukes or whether a lot of people in this county are dying that way."

"What do you mean, that way?"

"Dying not because they were so terribly injured, which a lot of them are, but because they just never got the care they needed in the hospitals where they were taken."

"And if you find out that people are dying like that, what are you going to be? A hero by going to 'Eyewitness News'?" She was looking at him, a touch of sarcasm playing in her eyes.

"Jesus Christ! What do you mean by that?" As surprised as he was he did not fail to realize that his response, which under other circumstances would have been marked by anger, was instead tinged with hurt.

"I mean, if you find out that a lot of people are dying because surgeons are off playing golf or sleeping with their favorite scrub

53

nurses, what are you going to do with the information?"

Allan shrugged. "I'm not really sure. From time to time, someone talks about the need for an official trauma center in San Francisco County, but it's all been vague."

"Why vague?"

"Because no one is really full-square for it. Some medical types have been saying we should have one because they have trauma centers in other places. But then everybody else is saying that medical care has traditionally been better in San Francisco County and besides the area is so small that no one is ever very far away from a hospital if there is an emergency."

"So now you want to find proof that there should be a trauma center?"

Allan felt uneasy. He dabbed with his fork for the remaining pieces of his burrito. "Anybody ever tell you you should have been a prosecuting attorney?"

"Hey," she shot back. "You came looking for me, and if you want my help, which you obviously do, then I want to know just what it is I'm helping with." He looked up at her and she broke into a laugh. "I guess I've just committed myself to at least thinking about helping you." She stopped, lifted her glass, never taking her eyes off him as she slowly drew on the beer. Allan met her gaze, feeling it more than seeing it. There was something unsettling in those eyes, with all the emotions they reflected. At times she seemed to be enjoying a private joke, her eyes reflecting a hint of self-satisfaction that, besides bringing a stirring between his legs, touched him in an unaccustomed way. But there was also a trace of something else, something he had seen time and again in the eyes of people waiting in emergency-room hallways while a friend or relative was being worked on behind closed doors. It was a look of part fear, part tragedy, part anger.

She put down the glass, crossed her arms on the table, and looked past him. "I didn't just call the University hospital out of professional dedication," she said finally.

Allan was startled. "You mean you were trying to tip us to something?"

"No, not in the way you're thinking of." She spoke carefully, as if struggling to suppress an urge to blurt out something she knew she shouldn't.

"We are supposed to call hospitals," she continued, "to let them know when their diagnosis of the cause of death of a patient is not right. But I'm the only one who does it; the others figure the hospitals don't give a shit unless you tell them the patient died of bubonic plague. Hell, maybe not even bubonic plague. Anyway, every once in a while I call, but only in certain cases . . ."

" . . . when someone has died in an accident," Allan finished for her. "Why?"

She remained silent, caught, it seemed to Allan, in an inner struggle. "I'm not really sure, I guess," Julie said finally. "I thought it might help some of the hospitals if people at the M.E.'s office finally started doing what they were supposed to. It didn't seem worthwhile to have the pathologists here go through all the trouble of doing a post and then not letting anyone know the results. It just seemed that the information should be of value to someone."

Allan studied her. He was convinced that she was lying. "Okay. You know . . . we know the medical examiner's office conducts autopsies where it suspects the true mechanism of death has gone undiagnosed. How can I use those cases to find out the extent to which hospitals are failing to treat trauma patients properly?" He was glad that his mind seemed to be functioning rationally again.

"Put together a study. Collect one hundred cases. See what our autopsy results are. See what the hospitals where the patients died reported as the cause of death. Figure out in how many cases the two determinations differed. If in a lot of cases the people at the hospitals think the patient died as a result of injuries that were not reparable but the pathologist's report in those cases says the death was due to wounds that could have been fixed, you'll have a pretty good idea that you are right."

"That would be okay, I guess. But no one is going to accept that as proof that there are problems out in the community."

It was Julie's turn to be puzzled. "Why the heck not, Allan?"

"Because the people who don't want to accept the fact that

the county needs a trauma center or that hospitals are not doing a good job will say that a pathologist's decision on a cause of death is based on a dead body, on a static situation. They'll say that the doctors and surgeons were dealing with a dynamic situation and that the care they gave the patient was determined by the way he looked when he was still alive."

"What would you need to make your case?"

"The medical records detailing the patient's care. If the pathologist's report says that the cause of death was preventable, and if I can see if the doctors did anything to get at the real cause of death, then I can determine whether or not the care was appropriate. In other words, what I need is something that will give me the ability to determine if the E.R. people understood what was going on and, if they did, that they were able to get surgical consults in to give definitive care. Can you just see hospitals letting me rummage through their medical records?"

"You don't have to ask the hospitals to let you see their records," she said matter-of-factly.

"What am I going to do, break into their record rooms in the dead of night?"

"No, you don't have to take up a life of crime. When we establish that we have to do an autopsy, we automatically request that the hospital send us all their records on the patient. E.R. records, O.R. records, records kept while the patient was on the floor. Even nurse's notes. By law, the hospitals have to comply."

Allan felt light-headed. "You have medical records on patients in your offices? I could see them?"

"Why not? We have researchers coming through all the time. As long as you don't violate the patient's—well, the deceased's—privacy, no one cares."

Allan slammed his fist down on the table and let out a whoop. Julie jumped back, alarmed then amused. "I'm glad you're so thrilled. But it won't be as easy as all that. There are about thirty thousand cases in our active file room and if you want to find your one hundred cases of trauma deaths, you're going to have to go through every file. That's a lot of suicides and murders and pneumonias and what have you to slog through."

"That's okay. When do we start?"

"We don't, friend. You do. It's your project, not mine. Anyway, you'll have to work after hours because there is just too much going on during the day, what with cops, lawyers, and God knows who else coming in to review files."

Allan thought for a moment, working out his decision. After hours meant after 5:30 P.M., even midnight in some cases, when he came off duty at the University and either went to one of the community hospitals for his moonlighting shift or home to get a few hours of sleep. If he undertook the study he would lose money, not to mention more sleep. But it didn't take him long to make up his mind. "Can I start tomorrow when I'm through with my shift?"

At six the following evening he was back at the morgue. He found his way into the parking lot through the gathering mist and walked to the double glass doors, his steps echoing off the pavement. He rang the bell and when the old security man opened the door he asked for Julie. A few minutes later she came for him.

She gave Allan a quick smile and a "Hi" and then led him down one of the long hallways out of the reception area. "Christ," he said, trying to make conversation, "it's as quiet as a morgue."

"All the bureaucrats have gone home," she said. "There'll be no one here except you, about two hundred stiffs in various stages of dissection, and one very old, very tired security man. If you hear any funny noises, don't panic."

He smiled at her, not sure if she was kidding or not. With a security key she opened the elevator door where they had stopped. They stepped in and she punched Basement.

When they entered the basement room that served as the repository for records, Allan felt sheer panic. To the left of the door, stretching from floor to ceiling, were fifty rows of file racks. The scene repeated itself to his right. He almost felt like crying. He would never have the time to go through all those cases and find the ones he was looking for. And, if somewhere in the recesses of his mind he was hoping that Julie would take pity on him and stay to help, he was soon disappointed. "Got a date," she said lightly. "Have fun. And don't get off on the wrong floor when you leave."

With that she was gone.

When, at two in the morning, he decided to call it quits, Allan was thoroughly depressed. After Julie had left him, he arbitrarily decided to start at the far right end of the files and work his way to the left. By the time he was ready to leave he had managed to make his way through only three of the file racks. He would be here for weeks, if not months, trying to find the cases that would fit his study.

The slow and tedious fashion in which he had to take each file off a shelf, mark the place where he had gotten it with a long strip of colored paper, look through its contents, and then put it back had not been the worst of the ordeal. More discouraging was that in the nearly seven hours of work he had found only one case that he could legitimately make a part of his study. As Julie had predicted, many of the files contained information about cases he was not interested in. When he did come across deaths that were due to accidents or stabbings and shootings, he had to pass them by for any number of reasons. Some because an autopsy had not been performed, probably because the medical examiner's office was chronically shorthanded. Others because, even if the autopsy had been done, the notes dictated by the medical examiner who had performed the postmortem had never been transcribed. He had to discard many other cases because the hospitals where the patients had been treated had, contrary to the law's requirements, not bothered to forward treatment records.

And, most of all, he found, his task was made immensely more difficult by the constant struggle to keep Julie off his mind. Wearily, he gathered his notes, put on his jacket, and headed for home.

The second, third, and fourth nights were unbearable. Each time, dressed in a new outfit, smelling fresh, looking vibrant, Julie greeted him with a broad, friendly smile and a few questions about the progress of his research. And, after leading him to the file room, she would leave him with a perky "Good night." He began to find more and more cases, and the growing pile of deaths should have brought him satisfaction. But somehow they didn't. As a surgeon, as someone who found life devoid of emergency surgeries a bore, the long hours of meticulous sorting through the files were torture. The tedium of his task was underlined by the gathering ache he felt for Julie and by his simmering resentment toward the offhand, noncommittal friendliness with which she treated him.

The fifth evening she lingered in the file room. Unsettled by the sudden change in the routine, not knowing what to say, Allan methodically began to arrange his papers, files, and pencils on the long conference table that occupied one corner of the room. He could feel her eyes on him.

"You're working too hard, you know, Allan," she finally said. "Have you looked in the mirror lately?"

"Young doctors are supposed to look like this. We wouldn't be credible if we didn't." Totally confused, unable to imagine where this conversation could go, he was determined to say no more than necessary.

"Well, I've seen stiffs that looked better than you do right now. Come on, Allan, let's go out. It won't kill you to let this go for one night. There's a county fair on in Santa Rosa. We can be there in an hour."

"Go to a county fair? Are you serious?"

"Yes, I'm very serious. Come on. I'll drive and it will be my treat."

He fought with himself, but it was a weak effort, and fifty-five minutes later Julie was at one of the ticket booths in front of the fairground's gates, buying admission tickets. Despite his skepticism, he soon found himself caught up in Julie's enthusiasm for the livestock displays and her determination to march up and down the aisles of the crowded, hot tents housing the homemade jams, jellies, and assorted other preserves. He followed her into the seats of tractors and combines and watched as young farm children fussed, for the last time, over livestock they would be entering in the various competitions and then selling at auction. And between each venture into each tent or display, he struggled to keep up as she dashed to buy dishes of barbecued beef, to gather samples of chili, to treat them to a pile of french-fried onion rings, to a plate of fresh corn drenched in butter.

None of which prepared him for what was to come. By the time Julie had polished off some freshly churned ice cream, they had come to the end of the farm and home-arts displays and had arrived at the entrance to the fair's carnival. The lights, the music, mixed with the cries and laughter of those people braving their terrors on the rides, broke over Julie and Allan. With a cry of delight, Julie grabbed Allan's hand, made for the first booth she saw, and bought a handful of tickets. Allan, totally in her power, squelched, not without difficulty, the desire to admit he had always been afraid of any ride wilder than a merry-go-round.

They began with the spinning saucers, then immediately made for a ride through a haunted house, a ride marked by sudden drops of their car and swift turns around ninety-degree corners. But for Julie these were obviously only warm-up events. In quick succession came trips on trains that traveled at right angles to the earth, in cars that spun and turned upside down, in a roller coaster, a double ferris wheel, a device in which the floor dropped away after centrifugal force had pinned the participants against the ride's walls. To Allan, the music and the noises seemed to grow louder each time he took his seat in yet another coach and had yet another ride attendant strap him in for another few minutes of unalloyed fright. After a while he even forgot that at first he had been charmed by Julie's enthusiasm for the thrills of the rides. By the time they went, at her insistence, for their second fling on a ride highlighted by a sign warning that pregnant women and people with heart conditions, high blood pressure, and a tendency to seizures should not partake, he was far beyond caring. Even survival was not uppermost in his mind. Only a chance to get to a bathroom and rid himself of all the foods they had eaten, foods he was only barely keeping down.

On the way back to San Francisco, Julie drove slowly, though Allan, now somewhat recovered, could not be sure whether she was doing so to savor the good time she had had or whether to prolong their time together. He leaned against the door and looked over at her. She was relaxed in the driver's seat, the fingers of one hand grasping the upper right side of the steering wheel, the fingers of the other hand resting lightly on the lower portion of the rim. In the soft light of the moon, her face seemed to glow with a quiet contentment. Allan wanted badly to reach over and caress her cheek, and started to raise his hand to carry out the impulse. But he wavered and did nothing. The rest of the trip dissolved into casual talk and, finally, a strange quiet. By the time Julie dropped him off in the medical examiner's parking lot so he could retrieve his car, he was thoroughly depressed. The outing may have done wonders for my coloring, he said to himself after they had said good night, but it hasn't done a thing for my morale.

The following evening, instead of merely unlocking the door to the file room and saying good night after a few perfunctory remarks, Julie followed him in and closed the door behind her.

"I've got nothing doing tonight," she said almost curtly. "Why don't I give you a hand for an hour or so?"

"Sure," he answered, trying to build some enthusiasm into his voice. "That would be terrific."

Julie looked at him, uncertainty in her eyes. She started to say something, but changed her mind. "How far have you gotten here?" she asked instead. "And where do you want me to start?"

With exaggerated politeness Allan showed her the stack he had finished the last time he had been in the room. "Why don't you start here," he said. "I'll go down to the other end and work from there toward you."

Allan moved away, cursing himself for his attitude, not knowing how to change it, how not to be petulant. As he worked from file to file, as he heard her movements at the other side of the room, he even had difficulty concentrating on his task because, as hard as he tried, he could not explain to himself exactly what he was being petulant about. Had he been hoping that the previous evening would end in bed? Was he angry because she was so much in control? More than that, was it because she seemed to have absolutely no need for him?

He was suddenly aware that she was yelling at him from the other side of the room. "Listen to this," she was saying excitedly. "Here's a forty-eight-year-old woman who rear-ends another car stopped for a red light, okay?"

Allan walked over, Julie continuing to read. "The paramedics take her to the E.R. at White Memorial. According to the E.R. notes, she is fully awake, talking coherently. Forty-five minutes later, the E.R. clerk starts to call the consults. Now listen to what it says in the clerk's notes:

"'Twelve-twenty A.M.: Dr. Alvarez called. Refused patient.

Suggested cardiac surgeon. Twelve-thirty A.M.: Dr. Garrison called. Refused case. Twelve-thirty-five A.M.: Dr. Eisen called. Could not be reached. Twelve-thirty-eight A.M.: Dr. Saticoy called. Suggested Dr. Mendelbaum. Twelve-forty A.M.: Dr. Mendelbaum called. Refused patient. Suggested a cardiologist. Twelve-fifty-five A.M.: Dr. Ashland called. Responded immediately. One A.M.: Patient lost consciousness. Dr. Ashland arrives one-ten A.M. Patient taken to ICU.'

"And that ain't all, folks," Julie went on. "The woman died in the ICU three hours later. The only thing that had been done for her was that she was given some fluids."

"And the autopsy says what?"

"She had a lacerated spleen."

"She bled to death from a simple, minimal injury, Julie. That woman should have been in and out of the operating room in an hour and a half and out of the hospital inside of a week."

Ten minutes later she called over again. "How about this one? Seventy-six-year-old guy, driving a car at about thirty miles an hour, runs a red light and smashes into a truck. They rush him to St. Luke's. One of the first things they do is run a blood test on him."

"That's all right. What'd they decide?"

Julie leafed through the papers, then laughed. "I'm sorry," she said, "I know it isn't funny, but . . . Yes, they did do a red-blood-cell count and it did come out abnormally low. But they decided it was because the old man was anemic. Then they shoved him into ICU."

"And he died, when?"

"Five hours later. According to the autopsy the cause of death was hemorrhaging secondary to a ruptured kidney."

The hour she had volunteered turned into two, then three. And while she was finding case after case for Allan's study, he also was having more luck. By the time midnight came and they decided to stop, the meager pile of a dozen cases Allan had managed to put together during his previous nights at the morgue had doubled to twenty-four.

As they walked out of the file room and made their way out of the silent building, Allan realized that his mood had dramatically improved. Not because he had made progress this time around, but because electricity had built up in the course of the evening.

"Want to stop somewhere for a drink?" he asked as they reached the front door.

"I thought you didn't drink because you might always be called in," she teased.

"That's not answering my question." He worked hard to sound matter-of-fact.

"I don't think so, thanks. It's late and I've got to be back here in eight hours. I want to get some sleep."

Allan couldn't contain himself. "What's the matter with you?" he yelled. "Why are you so goddamn standoffish, so damned—I don't know what. I mean, Christ!"

Julie regarded him with undisguised amusement. "You're not making too much sense, you know."

"Stop playing games. You know damned well what I mean."

"I guess I do, yes. But I'm taking you at your word, you know. That you came down here to do a study, not to establish a social life."

"I'm not trying to establish a social life, not that I've got much time for it. I enjoy your company, Julie. I just thought a drink to top off the evening would be nice."

"I'm sorry. But no."

Silently they walked through the parking lot to her car. She opened the door and turned to face him. Somehow the light mist seemed to soften her features even more, making it seem as if she would just simply melt away before him. Again, that urge to touch her swept through him. And again he kept one hand tightly wrapped around the handle of his briefcase, the other tucked tight in his pocket.

If Julie had noticed the emotion in his eyes she gave no hint of it. "I think you are doing something important here," she finally said, breaking the quiet. "And I want to help you with it. But I want you to understand that there won't be anything beyond that."

Allan said nothing.

"Do you have a deadline in mind for finishing?" she went on, refusing to be swayed by his air of hurt.

"I guess so. There's a meeting of the Joint Committee for Emergency Medical Services coming up pretty soon. I'd like to have the cases picked and analyzed by then."

"To present there?" There was open skepticism in her question.

"I don't know. Probably not. But at least I want to have that date as an objective."

"Well, if you decide you want me to help you, give me a call in the morning. I'll be in by eight." And with that she was in her car and starting the engine. But before she could engage the gear shift, Allan reached in and took hold of the steering wheel.

"Why the sudden interest in my work, McDonough?" he asked. "It can't be because you're so convinced that I'm doing something important."

She looked directly at him. "Nothing is going on, Dr. Kirk. You're giving me a chance to work on something that has muscle and blood to it, not just a bunch of numbers. I'm taking the opportunity, that's all. Don't be so paranoid, I'm not an undercover agent for the hospital association." She put the car in gear and drove off almost before he had a chance to withdraw his arm.

Allan watched her drive slowly out of the parking lot. You're no spy, he said to himself. But you're not being completely honest with me either.

4

The sun, in its swing toward the west, was on the other side of the Golden Gate Bridge. Its rays on this unusually warm day played on the bridge's two great towers, bringing their red coloring to a fireplace-glow intensity. A sailboat, taking full advantage of the brisk wind whipping and snapping into the bay, coursed beneath the structure, cutting smartly through its shadows silhouetted on the waters.

Up on the long stretch of green grass running parallel to the water, the part of San Francisco the city residents know as Marina Green Park, two joggers huffed and puffed their way past the scores of sunbathers, the picnicking families, a lone flute player practicing his repertoire, and four volleyball games where dozens of young men and women were playing or cheering enthusiastically.

Because the woman jogger was listening to a tape of Beethoven's *Eroica* Symphony on her portable cassette player, the man running with her reached out, tapped her on the shoulder, and nodded to their right. She nodded back, and, in perfect timing, the two turned and sped off across the broad expanse of green toward Marina Boulevard. They stopped at the curb—though they kept their legs pumping—and in response to another unspoken signal began their dash across the boulevard when the way seemed clear. With a laugh she picked up speed, clearly wanting to make a race of it.

The Buick, its tires squealing as it pulled out of a parking place 150 feet down the block, was upon them in an instant. Because she had opened some distance between herself and the man, the automobile missed the woman. But its massive grill caught the man squarely, hurling him five feet into the air, ten feet down the street. He crashed into a van parked at the sidewalk, bounced back into the street, and came to rest in a heap, arms and legs pointed at odd angles. The portion of his body below his hips lay flat on the street. His abdomen and chest were twisted to the right. His head leaned forward, his chin touching his chest. The woman ran back to him and kneeled at his side. Her hands moved to his head, to his chest, back toward his head, almost as if she were administering a silent blessing meant to make him whole again.

The keening of the ambulance's siren parted the silent crowd that had gathered around the shattered jogger. Two young men leaped out of the van. One ran to the jogger, the other to the back of the ambulance to retrieve the large trauma box containing their medical instruments. On his return he spotted an elderly man at the edge of the crowd and asked him to draw the woman aside and comfort her.

The paramedic whose I.D. tag on his shirt identified him as Eric Drake leaned close to the jogger's head. A massive bruise ran along the right side of the man's face. Blood was running out of his ear. One eye was swollen shut.

"Is my wife all right?" the man mumbled.

"Fine. She's fine," Drake answered. "Just take it easy, we'll get you to a hospital in five minutes."

Working methodically, exchanging only a few words here and there, Drake and his colleague placed a cervical collar around the jogger's neck, then quickly measured his blood pressure. "Arnie, I'm going to call the base station and find out where we should take this guy," Drake said. "We've gotta get him in somewhere quick."

Drake ran to the van. Within two minutes he was back.

"Where do we take him?" Arnie asked.

"Coit Hill said to go nowhere. They want to dispatch the chopper."

"I guess that gives us some time to really stabilize him."

"It doesn't give us any time. Waiting for the chopper is a bunch of horseshit. On one call last week it took them half an hour to get the crew organized and get their toy off the ground. This guy's as good as dead. We can't wait for those fuckers."

"Then what are we going to do?"

"Take him to the U."

"I don't know, Eric. If the base station says to wait . . . We can stabilize him enough to hold him till they get here."

"No way. A case like this is too unpredictable. We're going to the University. It's probably the only shot this cat's got."

Reluctantly, Arnie went along. The two paramedics gently showed the still shaking woman to the ambulance, helped her in, then drew a backboard out of the vehicle. They ran back to the jogger, placed him on the backboard, and slid him into the ambulance. Drake took the wheel. His partner stepped into the back of the van, next to the jogger.

"Hey, Eric," Arnie shouted a few minutes later as they sped down Van Ness. "How are we going to explain disregarding instructions from a base station?"

"We don't have to explain. We sort of lost contact."

"What do you mean, sort of? How can you sort of lose contact?"

"You can if the radio goes dead on you while you're talking to the base station."

"You hung up on the doc?" Arnie screeched.

"Not quite. But, see, there's this loose wire on the radio I've been meaning to tell maintenance to repair. Gosh, while I was talking to the base station I reached down there to make sure it was working. And damned if it didn't come apart completely. Just when the doc was asking me to repeat this guy's vital signs and to tell him exactly where we were at the Marina and where they should land."

"We're going to be in deep shit if Anthony hears about it and doesn't buy it," Arnie said with a nervous laugh.

"Fuck Anthony. Fuck Coit Hill. And fuck that new bronze Trauma Treatment Center sign they planted on the front lawn. It may take us another three minutes to get to the University. But at least it won't take them an hour and a half to get a surgeon in. I'll worry about Anthony another day, Arnie. How's our friend doing?"

"His blood pressure is dropping. I can hardly palpate it. His pulse is weaker and thready. I've got two liters of Ringer's lactate going in wide open."

"Well, hang on. We should be there in a minute." Drake increased the volume of their siren and stepped down harder on the accelerator.

As he hustled down the corridor to the meeting room, Allan unwrapped the clinging cellophane from the sandwich he had grabbed off a shelf in the cafeteria. He crunched the wrapping into a tight ball, flipped it into an ashtray standing near a bank of elevators, and took a massive bite out of the turkey, lettuce, and wheat-bread combination. Trying to collect his thoughts for the seminar he was about to lead for some of the new residents, he was only dimly aware of the wail of the distant ambulance. But as the high-pitched sound grew louder and louder, he stopped, then ran to a nearby house phone.

"That for us?" he asked when the emergency-room desk clerk had answered.

"No idea, Dr. Kirk. No one has called us about an incoming. Maybe it's just a cardiac."

"Maybe." Allan hung up, took another bite from his sandwich, and started again toward the seminar. But after a few steps, he changed his mind, stuffed the rest of the sandwich into his mouth, and, chewing rapidly, ran down to the emergency room. He moved past several nurses toward the double doors giving onto the receiving dock where the ambulances stopped to drop off their patients. Just as he stepped out into the fresh air, the ambulance swept down the broad driveway and braked to a halt in front of him.

The van's back door flew open and Allan stepped forward to look inside.

"Holy shit, Drake," Allan said when the paramedic had reached him. "This guy looks like he's ready to code. Why didn't you give us a call?"

"Tried to, doc," Drake said, doing his best to look embarrassed. "But the goddamn radio's been giving us trouble all day. It conked out on us just as we took off to get here."

"What have you got?"

"A jogger who was creamed by a car. We brought in his wife, too. But she's okay," Drake said as he helped the jogger's wife out of the ambulance, then turned to help Arnie and Allan pull on the backboard with the unconscious jogger.

"What are his vital signs?" Allan asked as they put the jogger on a gurney and pushed it toward the emergency-room doors.

"Deteriorating. Blood pressure at the scene was 40/0 but we got it back to 80/40 with fluids. On the way in it crashed. All he's got is a thready pulse," Drake answered.

"Okay, let's get him into the trauma room before he arrests on us. I'll have one of the residents look after his wife and try to find out more about him."

Allan, the two paramedics, and Joe Santorre, the senior resident, who had now joined them on the receiving dock, propelled the gurney at top speed into the trauma room. Running alongside the patient, Allan placed his hand close to his mouth, then glanced down to his chest.

"He breathing, Kirk?" Santorre asked.

"Not adequately."

Even before they had come to a full stop inside, the trauma team anesthesiologist positioned himself at the head of the gurney. Using a laryngoscope, he opened the jogger's mouth and quickly sucked out blood, mucus, and shards of broken teeth. "Airway's clear," he called out to Allan.

"Okay, but let's put in an endotracheal tube and bag him; he'll need all the help possible to get those lungs expanded."

As a nurse whipped a blood pressure cuff onto the jogger's right arm, another nurse and an intern, each wielding giant scissors, made short work of the man's jogging pants, his shirt, and an elastic bandage covering most of his left thigh.

"Blood pressure down to 40/20," one of the nurses called out.

"I've got him intubated and his lungs are expanding, but this guy's got some big problems, let me tell you," the anesthesiologist chimed in, the rhythm of his words timed to the rhythm with which he was squeezing and releasing the oxygen bag connected to a tube leading into the jogger's mouth.

"Type and cross him for twelve units of blood," Allan called out. "Notify the O.R. Tell them we'll be up in ten minutes, if not sooner. Get a big-bore IV in each arm." Allan paused and looked around. "Brooks, get a cut-down going in the right ankle."

Maggie Brooks, the young physician who a day earlier had been assigned to the trauma team for two months as part of her rotating internship program, turned to the instrument table to find the cut-down tray. Allan returned his attention to the jogger.

"For starters we have a potential head injury," Allan now began to recite, to give the entire team an inventory of the jogger's probable injuries. "Severe contusion around the right temple, blood trickling from right ear. Patient is now unresponsive. Drake said his pupils were equal in the field but the right one is now widely dilated and unresponsive."

"I'd say you got hemorrhaging into the right side of the brain," Santorre interrupted.

"I'd say you're right, we're going to have to two-team this guy," Allan said, never taking his eyes off the jogger as his hands skated over the surface of the man's body. "Rib fractures on both sides." He slipped on his stethoscope. "Diminished breath sounds. Let's get set up for bilateral chest tubes."

"X rays, doctor?" one of the nurses asked.

"No. We'll do just one to make sure the chest tubes are in place before he goes to the O.R. That's about all we'll have time for."

Allan moved down the side of the gurney. "Distended abdomen, pelvis unstable," he continued out loud. "Fractures of the extremities, the femur on the right leg, tibia and fibula on the left. Color of legs is good, pulses not bad." Allan looked up. "Harris, do the rectal," he said to an intern who had just come on the scene.

"What do you think, Kirk?" Santorre asked as he began to cut into the left side of the jogger's chest in order to place the tube that would drain away the loose blood accumulating on the right side of the man's thorax.

Busily cutting into the other side of the inert body to provide access for a tube into the chest, Allan shook his head just slightly. "If this guy makes it, it will be a miracle."

"Hell, we've seen worse," Santorre said, his voice strained by his effort to push his tube, which he had already inserted into the cut, farther into the chest cavity.

"Don't think so," Allan said, reaching over to an instrument table to locate a chest tube. "If we go according to the injury-severity-score concept and total up the points for the chest injury, the epidural hemorrhage, and so on, I'd say we'd reach an eighty-six as an index. We've saved a seventy-five and I think an eighty. But I've never seen anyone with an injury-severity score this high make it. He'll be lucky to make it out of the O.R."

Allan looked up and saw that the portable X-ray machine had been brought to the jogger's bedside. "All right, let's get that placement film. And let's get the Foley catheter in and drain his bladder. Get a nasogastric tube in. I don't want this guy aspirating his vomit on the O.R. table."

"Should we prep for a peritoneal lavage?" a nurse hooking up another two liters of Ringer's lactate asked.

"No point in it," Allan answered, now stitching the chest tube in place with a heavy silk suture, "Let's not waste the time. Santorre, your tube yield anything?"

"About eight hundred cc's. Yours?"

Allan looked beneath the bed at the bottle connected to the chest tube he had inserted. "About two hundred. Blood pressure?"

"He's drifting back down again. I can barely hear it at sixty," the nurse monitoring the jogger's pulse said.

"Get him more fluids," Allan said, anxiety in his voice now. "Brooks, you got anything going into that ankle cut-down yet?"

There was no answer.

Allan spun toward the jogger's feet. Maggie Brooks was still bent over the man's ankle. He could see sweat glistening on her forehead like a delicate string of beads just under her hairline. And yet, though she looked as if she had been laboring hard, she had not yet finished cutting through the skin.

"Come on, damnit. You're not cutting a pattern for a dress," he said, immediately regretting the remark.

He moved toward her. "Look, the skin is thick. You've got to put pressure on that knife. Just push down, nice and easy," he said, soothingly. "Imagine you're cutting into a hunk of cheddar cheese at a party."

Though there was a slight tremor in Maggie's hand, the scalpel disappeared farther into the jogger's ankle. Allan could feel her tension.

"Now take the mosquito clamp and probe the incision for the vein," he said quietly, as if he were talking her through nothing more crucial than minor stitchwork on a three-inch cut in a youngster's arm. But he could see her jaws working, her lips grow tauter, whiter.

She probed. Probed again. Now, using more force, she jammed the clamp deep into the incision.

He grabbed her hand. She released the clamp and moved back. With two or three quick flicks of the wrist, he separated the fat and brought the cordlike white saphenous vein into view. A nurse offered him a thick tube. He took it, nicked the vein, slipped the tube through the small cut into the hollow of the vessel, then tied the tube in place.

"Okay, run that IV wide open," he said as he straightened up. He saw that a nurse was opening the valve controlling the flow of the Ringer's lactate into the jogger's ankle. Maggie's surgical cap lay crumpled on an instrument tray. But Maggie Brooks was gone.

He shrugged and looked at the clock. Eight minutes had passed since the jogger had been brought through the E.R. doors.

"We've got a tube in his nose and he's catheterized. His chest X ray looks okay. His urine output is low." Santorre was talking in measured tones, letting his voice tell Allan that he did not approve of the time Allan had taken with the inept intern.

"The O.R. just called," a nurse chimed in. "The neuro-surgeon is up there, but he's not too happy about going in without a CAT scan."

"He'll have to live with it," Allan answered. "Let's get going."

Santorre and Allan positioned themselves at the foot of the bed. Two interns and two first-year trauma residents jockeyed for positions at the jogger's side. The nurses stood at the head of the bed, one at each side of the anesthesiologist. The interns and residents grabbed fluid bottles and blood bags. Then, as if they had all been standing behind a racetrack gate that had suddenly been flung open, they began to run.

Pirouetting, twisting, skipping sideways, they squeezed through doors, hurled themselves and their patient down narrow hallways, negotiated their way around tight corners, only to come to a skidding halt at the elevator doors.

Allan pushed a button, the doors opened. In almost perfect synchronization, the nurses and physicians took deep breaths and squeezed close against the gurney so they could all push into the elevator. There was a sound of clashing glass as the front wheels of the gurney passed over the threshold, jangling the fluid bottles on their stands. Twisting to reach past one of the nurses, an intern lifted the stands, then lowered them to draw them into the elevator. With a heave, the anesthesiologist lifted the back of the gurney, freeing the rear wheels, which had twisted and caught in the space between the elevator and the hall floor. Now Allan and the others stared malevolently at the doors, wondering in silence why they had to close so excruciatingly slowly, while the patient edged closer to death.

Almost as slowly, the elevator left the ground and made its way to the second floor. Two nurses and the anesthesiologist, who had come into the elevator last and who were therefore closest to the door, inched forward in anticipation. With a long, mournful sigh, the elevator crept to a stop. After a second's pause, the doors began their slow-motion effort to open. With a whispered "God-damn stupid elevators," the anesthesiologist squeezed through and, like a football lineman trying to open a gap in the opposing team's defenses, forced the doors wider apart.

The team and the gurney spilled out and sped the last fifty feet to the operating room.

They brought the gurney to a stop within inches of the operating table. Interns and nurses scrambled to sort out and untangle the half-dozen intravenous tubes leading into the jogger's arms and legs. One resident quickly checked the chest tubes to make sure they were secure. A nurse adjusted the thin tube leading into the jogger's nose.

"Watch his pecker," Santorre said to no one in particular. "The last thing we need is that Foley pulling out and bringing the prostate with it."

"Come on, come on," Allan called out. "Let's get him on the table. Ready? One, two . . ."

At the count of three, they heaved and in one swift motion placed the jogger on the operating table.

"Blood pressure, blood pressure!" Allan yelled, glancing again at the clock, seeing that now fifteen minutes had elapsed since the jogger arrived downstairs.

"I can't get a blood pressure," a nurse shot back.

"Pulse."

"He's got a barely palpable carotid pulse," another female voice called out.

"We don't have time to scrub up," Allan said. "Pour some Betadine solution over his chest and belly."

"He's running on oxygen alone right now, Kirk," the anesthesiologist interrupted. "When you're ready to go in I'll give you some muscle paralysis."

"You going to have to give him any gas?" Allan asked.

"The shape he's in, we can't give him anything. Don't worry, if he makes it he's not going to remember a thing."

A nurse grabbed a bottle of Betadine, tore off its cap, and emptied the reddish-brown disinfectant on the naked body. Another nurse reached for the instrument table, found a razor, and, in a single, smooth motion, cut through the thick, golden curly hair on the man's chest and abdomen, leaving behind a naked strip of skin, a ribbon that cut from the Adam's apple to the pubic bone like a straight Iowa road through miles of cornfields. Allan put on his gown, a mask, and gloves, then threw sterile drapes over the jogger's genitals and legs, and ran one drape across the neck to separate the head from the rest of the body.

Dimly aware that the neurosurgeon had begun shaving the jogger's head, Allan picked up his scalpel.

"Doctor," one of the nurses called out, "please give us a

minute to set up our instruments and get the lights adjusted."

Allan motioned for Santorre, who would be acting as his first assistant, to take his position across from him, then looked to the anesthesiologist to make sure he was ready. The man gave a thumbs-up sign.

Allan took the scalpel and with two long, quick strokes was into the abdominal cavity. Simultaneously, Santorre and the other resident put their hands into the gaping wound and pulled the two sides of flesh up and away. Allan took two more swipes with his scalpel then jerked it back as the abdominal cavity opened fully, pouring blood out onto the table. The high-pitched whine of a drill sounded as the neurosurgeon started to cut into the jogger's skull.

Allan reached into the belly and grabbed the aorta at the point where it enters the upper abdomen, underneath the diaphragm, and pinched it to redirect more blood to the jogger's upper body and brain.

"Pressure is coming up," the anesthesiologist said. "I've got a reading of sixty systolic."

"Good. I'm going to cross-clamp the aorta and leave it for a few minutes while you put some more blood into him." Allan looked back down at the jogger. "Get me a basin quickly," he said to a nurse, "the belly's still full of blood."

A basin materialized at his side. He reached into the belly and pulled out large gelatinous clumps of clots the size of grapefruits.

Taking white sterile cloth packs from a scrub nurse, Allan pushed them into the cavity. Save for the sound of the machine the neurosurgeon was using to suction blood and fluids from inside the jogger's skull, there was quiet in the operating room as Allan bent over to do a step-by-step inventory of the damage wrought by the Buick.

"What we are dealing with here," Allan said after a silence of two minutes, "is a shattered spleen, a massive liver injury, multiple perforations in the bowel, retroperitoneal hemorrhage with possible injury to kidney or pancreas, a massive pelvic hematoma."

"Well, there goes my dinner date," Santorre said. "Retractor, please."

The nurse handed him the instrument. He placed its curved

edges on one side of the abdominal cavity and pulled hard.

Allan reached deep into the abdomen with his left hand, brought up the spleen, and clamped off blood vessels running to it. With a few snips of his surgical scissors, he cut it free. With barely a second look, he handed it to the scrub nurse, who dropped the organ into the basin she was holding. Allan made a mental note to tell the family that he would be able to live without the spleen, but because the organ helped the body with its immunological response to some bacteria, he would always be at higher risk for infections.

"Pressure?"

"Up to one-ten. Looking better."

"How many units of blood has he used?"

"He's up to sixteen units."

"All right. Give him two more units and let me know when they're in. I want to get this clamp off the aorta as soon as possible."

Allan put his hand back into the belly and brought up several loops of bowel that had been perforated.

"I'm just going to cross-clamp the area of the perforation to stop more shit from coming out," Allan said to Santorre. "I'll get back to it later. We'd better control the bleeding from the liver first."

Allan took a retractor from the nurse on his left and handed it to the resident acting as his second assistant. "I know you can't see what's going on, but we're going to need your strength. Give me steady traction on that retractor."

When the resident had pulled the edge of the abdominal incision back as far as possible, Allan took out the packs he had earlier placed around the liver. Blood welled up quickly from the deep and jagged cracks on the surface of the liver.

"Put some fresh packs on that, will you, Santorre, while I cross-clamp its blood supply."

Allan removed the packs Santorre had just placed. Blood continued to pour out of the crevices. He turned to Santorre. "We've got a big problem. The bleeding is at the level of the vena cava. If I lift the right lobe of the liver so I can get a shot at it, we'll open up the tear and he'll bleed out in two minutes."

"What are you going to do?" Santorre asked.

"I'm going to go in from above. Let's open the chest."

Using first a scalpel, he cut the jogger's skin from the top of the sternum to where the abdominal incision started. Then, taking the sternal saw, he cut through the breastbone, exposing the heart and its great vessels. The jogger was open from his neck to his pubic bone. Allan inserted a thumb-sized tube through the wall of the heart's right upper chamber and threaded the tube into the major vein leading past the liver. He placed a tourniquet on the vein itself so that blood coming from the lower part of the body was diverted into the tube and bypassed the liver. Now Allan, without fearing that he would trigger a hemorrhage, moved the large organ. He saw the blood vessels attaching the liver to the inferior vena cava and spotted the tear in the thick blood vessel.

"Retract the liver for me, Santorre," he called out.

Santorre pulled the liver back and Allan, with wrist movements that would have done an Eastern European seamstress proud, whipped stitches through the vena cava, closing the laceration.

"There," Allan finally said. "Got the son of a bitch!"

Allan straightened up slowly, trying to ease away the tension that had built up in his lower back. "Going to have to start doing some back exercises or one of these days I'll never straighten up again. How are his vitals?"

"Blood pressure is 80/60, pulse is one-twenty," the anesthesiologist answered. "Considering how long we've had to work on him, he's not doing badly and is holding his own. But we've already used twenty-four pints of blood. I wouldn't spend too much more time in there if I were you."

"What about his head?"

For a moment the neurosurgeon, concentrating on closing the bony flap he had opened in the jogger's skull, did not respond. "He had a beaut of an epidural hemorrhage," he finally answered. "Five more minutes of bleeding like that and it would have been bye-bye. But he's responded well."

"Fine. But I still have to tidy up the injuries to the bowel, do a temporary colostomy, and do some more sewing on the liver. Can you hold him that long?"

"Okay," the anesthesiologist answered. "But I wouldn't push my luck, Kirk."

Allan, hypnotized by his work, soothed by the Willie Nelson someone had slipped into the tape deck in the corner of the room, worked for an hour and a half without looking up.

"I think we've done just about all we can," he said when he had taken the last stitch into the liver. He turned to Santorre. "Finish up, would you? Irrigate him, put some drains in, and close up. And don't forget to set him up for some platelets. Make sure you get a check on his clotting factors."

"You going to see if the woman that was with him is up to talking?"

"Thought I would, yes. If she's not, I hope they found some other relatives." Allan headed for the door, then stopped. "We have any whole blood left?"

"Two pints, doctor," answered one of the circulating nurses, whose job it was to do everything from obtaining additional supplies from the storeroom to calling the surgeon's stockbroker to get price quotes.

"Better than nothing, I guess. Take them back to the bank, would you?"

The circulating nurse, an unspoken plea immediately visible in her eyes, exchanged glances with two other nurses. Neither one of them said a word.

"Okay, what is it now?" Allan asked, sensing something was amiss.

"We can't do it, doctor," the circulating nurse said, but not before casting an if-looks-could-kill glance at the colleagues who had refused to come to her aid. "We still don't have the blood cooler. They have to be discarded."

Allan stepped back into the surgical suite. "I don't believe it! That'll make it ten units of blood we've had to piss away this week alone!"

Allan snatched the plastic bags containing the two units of blood and stormed out of the surgical suite, bloodstained greens and all. He half-walked, half-ran down the long hall to the elevators. Then, unwilling to wait for one to reach the floor, he stalked to the staircase, threw open the door, and climbed the stairs, taking two steps at a time, slapping at the rail every time he brought his hand down to grab it.

On the fourth floor he flung open the exit door and, now under a full head of steam, charged into the suite of the medical center's chief administrator. "Dr. Kirk, Mr. White is very . . . ," the administrator's secretary began as Allan roared past her and through the door leading into the administrator's office.

The man, who had been concentrating on some papers on his desk, looked up surprised. He opened his mouth to speak, but Allan, slamming the bags of blood on the papers, didn't give him a chance.

"How long have I been pleading with you for a blood cooler, Jack? Six months, eight months? You seem to find money for everything but a diddly little blood cooler."

"Allan, I've told you, the—" White answered, coming to his feet.

"Yeah, I know. The check is in the mail. Do you know what we have to go through to get enough blood stocked for surgeries?" Allan's voice rose. "Do you listen to the radio, Jack? Do you? Do you hear the constant appeals for blood, Jack, can you even guess how many of these babies we've had to throw away in the last six months because you can't get around to getting us a blood cooler?"

White, trying to escape Allan's anger, looked down at his desk and promptly turned pale. Allan sprang forward and just managed to grab White's lapels to help ease his crash into his chair. When Allan looked at the desk he saw that the bags had split open and were releasing their contents over White's work.

"You'd better see to your boss," Allan said to the secretary as he walked out past her. "I think he's fainted."

She scrambled out from behind her desk and ran into the office.

Feeling better, Allan slowly made his way back to the emergency room and asked for the jogger's wife. He found her in one of the treatment cubicles, sitting on the edge of the bed. Allan could see that she was still struggling to bring her emotions under control. Her blonde hair was only partly held together in its ponytail. In front, some of it spilled over her sweatband, now slightly askew. Narrow red streaks ran downward from her eyes.

"How are you feeling?" Allan asked softly.

She shrugged. "I don't know. Okay, I guess. Dizzy." She stopped and looked down. Allan knew she was struggling to ask about her husband without breaking down.

"Is he going to make it?" she asked in a whisper.

Allan sat down on the bed next to her and took her hand. "It's too early to tell," he said, soothingly. "He has some major injuries and he's going to need all the luck or prayers he can get."

Still looking at her knees, she began to sob quietly. "We've got two kids, one three years, one six months old." She paused, bit her lower lip. "Oh, God, what are we going to do?"

Her shoulders shook as she struggled to stifle her crying. Allan stroked her hand. When she began searching for a handkerchief she obviously did not have, he reached to the lower shelf of the bedstand and brought out the box of tissues that had been standing there. She wiped her eyes, freed her hand from Allan's grasp, stood up, and took a few steps away from the bed. She was tall, almost willowy, and had the posture and muscular legs of a well-trained athlete. She was steeling herself, preparing to ask the difficult questions. When she was ready, she moved back to the bed and sat down again. Allan gave her an exact accounting of her husband's injuries.

"What are his chances?" she asked when Allan was finished.

"I can't tell you that for another forty-eight or seventy-two hours. He seems to be in good physical shape and that means he's got something going for him. In any case, it's too early to tell."

She bent her head as her eyes began to moisten again.

"Have you called anyone?" Allan asked.

"My mother when we first got here. She was looking after the kids while we were out running. Doctor, what if he does survive, is it going to have to be with the help of machines? He wouldn't want that."

"If he lives through the next three days, it won't come to that. He'll have to work hard, you'll have to work hard, but there is no reason he couldn't in time be as productive as he ever was."

She nodded, a slow, ambiguous movement that told Allan that she did not quite believe him. "Can I see him now?"

"He's probably in the recovery room by now," Allan answered. "I'll take you in for five minutes, but please understand that he'll look terrible, even worse than he really is."

As they came to the wooden doors with their small windows and their large Authorized Personnel Only sign, Allan grew apprehensive. For a moment he considered asking her to wait another hour or two until they had had a chance to move him into an intensive-care-unit bed. But she was anxious and he decided to go ahead.

The jogger lay nude on a table at the far end of the room. Both legs and one arm, held fast by traction machinery, jutted up and away from the still body. A large white turban covered his head down to his eyebrows. His eyes were swollen shut. His face, like the rest of him, was puffy and pasty white. A long surgical bandage covered the massive incision. Around the incision, the cuts and bruises caused by the impact with the automobile were still highlighted by blood, dirt, and even small bits of glass. His chest, his nose, his penis, the crooks of his arms gave rise to a bewildering assortment of tubes. One large tube, pushing against a corner of his mouth, was connected to a ventilator standing by the side of the bed. His chest moved up and down in rhythm with the machine's quiet murmurings.

Allan, who had his arm around the woman's shoulder, felt her falter. "Would you rather wait?"

"No!" she answered fiercely. Slipping from his grasp, she moved to the bed. She put her hand lightly on the jogger's hand and bent over to kiss his eyes. "Bob," she cried quietly. "Don't die on me. Please don't die."

With some effort Allan managed to pry her away and out of the recovery room. Though he tried to convince her that there was nothing more she could do at the hospital for the moment, she insisted on staying. Allan showed her to a small waiting room and helped her to a chair. He'd better ask a nurse to look in on her, Allan said to himself.

He began to head for the elevators, then changed his mind. Though he longed to go home, he wanted to look in on the jogger once more.

Santorre came to meet him at the door. "I'm glad you came

back. We're not doing too well here. He just started giving indications that he's got a good case of red-ink syndrome going. He's oozing blood everywhere. His ears, the nose, the areas around the cut-downs, the abdominal incision. The works."

Allan stooped to look at the bottle receiving the jogger's urine. The liquid there was tinted red as well. "We must have gotten some bank blood even poorer than usual in clotting factors," he said. "You order the fresh frozen plasma yet?"

"Yeah. But they still haven't gotten here. Nor the platelets."

"When they do, just pour them in and order more. This guy's going to have a stormy course tonight, so stick with him. Keep a close eye on his blood gases, his clotting parameters, his urine output. Call me at home if he starts to sour."

Walking slowly to his car, allowing a gentle breeze to refresh his spirits, Allan spied a familiar figure just ahead of him.

"Maggie!" he called out. "What got into you up there?" he asked as he walked up. "That was not very professional behavior."

"I'm sorry if you think that being able to do a cut-down in forty-five seconds is the hallmark of professionalism," Maggie countered, refusing to be contrite.

"That's not what I mean and you know it. Why did you stomp out like that? Did you feel that you didn't have a responsibility to the patient?"

"Yes, I felt my responsibility to the patient. But I certainly did not feel it to you people." Maggie wheeled and walked away.

"What?" Allan was genuinely puzzled. It took him a moment to realize she was moving away from him at a fair clip. He started after her.

"You're all so goddamn smug on that trauma team, like you are the only ones in the whole medical universe qualified and able to fight death to a standstill." She was stalking now, not bothering to look at him striding at her side. "The truth is you could train a monkey to do resuscitation. You can take any mediocre technician and train him to start IVs, do cut-downs, do chest tubes. Big deal."

He reached out and stopped her. "Come on, wait a second,"

he said, trying to keep a light tone. "I can't talk and train for the Boston Marathon at the same time."

Maggie stopped and turned to face him. Working to muster as much contempt as possible into her stance, she contemplated him silently for a second. Then, her jet-black eyes flashing, she was off on another tirade. "In fact, I don't even know that there is a worthwhile intellectual challenge in being a surgeon, and the trauma surgeon is the least intellectually challenged of all. You take out a hundred spleens a year, sew up a couple of livers, and you think you should be ranked right up there with Jonas Salk. But you are nothing but big egos surviving with very little brains!" And with that she walked off again.

Though Allan was very sure that he should be angry with the upstart intern, he found that he could not muster very much bile against the young woman stomping farther and farther away from him. He thought for a couple of seconds, then trotted after her, catching her just as she came to her bus stop.

"Okay," he said, "now that you've gotten it off your chest, do you want to talk about it?"

"I don't know what you're talking about." She fished in the pocket of her white coat, looking for the exact change she would need for the bus.

"What I'm talking about is that while that was a very nice little speech, there's something bugging you about being on the service and whatever it is it has nothing to do with my monumental ego."

Rather than respond, Maggie stepped out into the street to see if her bus was coming yet. "Like it or not," Allan went on when she still refused to answer, "you are going to have to put in two months with us. Now you don't have to love me or even like me or Santorre or any of the other trained monkeys on the team. But the hard fact is that unless we work out what's bugging you, your attitude is going to kill a patient."

"There's nothing bugging me." Her tone was sullen, but her shoulders, he saw, had loosened up.

"Listen, have you had dinner yet?" he asked.

"In that ptomaine pit the med center has the nerve to call a cafeteria? Are you kidding?"

"See? There are worse things in the world than trauma surgeons."
She repressed a smile.

"Look," he went on. "Come have dinner with me. I'll cook you a Chinese meal you'll never forget."

An hour later, after a hectic chase through three Chinatown markets for eggplant, shrimp, pork, heavy soy sauce, ginger, garlic, chili paste, Chinese cabbage, red wine vinegar, and yellow onions, Allan was at his butcher block cutting, chopping, and mincing. Maggie, glass of wine in hand, was sitting on the counter next to the sink, watching him. If she was not pretty, Allan had decided earlier, she was certainly fascinating. Her eyes, when not expressing anger, shone with effervescence. Her curly black hair, her small, pert nose, and her almost too-small mouth gave her a doll-like appearance. She tilted her face slightly whenever he said something that genuinely seemed to interest her.

"So that's how you practice your skills," she teased, eyeing the cleaver as he moved it up and down with rapid wrist motions.

"No, that's the productive way in which I express my hostilities. You may think I'm cutting vegetables here but what I'm doing is slicing administrators who give me grief because my patients occupy beds too long. I'm cutting apart chiefs of staff who nag at me to reduce the number of people I have on the team, I'm making short work of interns who moralize after having been on the service for two hours. Very therapeutic."

"From talk around the center, I gather you could use a lot more therapy."

Allan laughed. He arranged the ingredients for the eggplant dish on one side of the butcher block, the ingredients for the hot shrimp on the other side. "Maybe," he said, as he turned the heat on under the wok and poured oil into it along the sides. "But my human targets generally deserve it when I land on them."

"Meaning that trauma surgeons, blessed souls they are, don't deserve the kind of judgments I make?"

He tossed the minced garlic into the now hot oil and stirred it, spreading it over the surface of the wok.

"No. Meaning more that you are making incomplete judgments...." He concentrated on stirring in the eggplant and ground pork, more spices, and a generous helping of sherry. For two minutes, as he stirred and moved the mixture of food around, there was silence.

"I don't know that they are incomplete judgments. The whole atmosphere around the E.R. and the trauma room is so sterile, so darned impersonal, it drives you up the wall. I hated my two months on the E.R. service just as much."

"I don't understand that at all. That's one of the services interns find the most exciting." He set out two dishes, chopsticks, a bottle of soda water for himself, the bottle of wine for Maggie.

"I'm saying it again. Because it's impersonal. It's like . . . ," she paused for a moment, searching for the right analogy. "Being in the E.R. is like being on a never-ending series of blind dates. With every patient you start all over again. You wonder if they like you. You wonder if they trust you. You know they are wondering if you're the woman who got into med school under a quota or if you were the one who had to go to some mill abroad to get your degree. You have to prove yourself over and over again. It's so depressing."

She stopped and poured herself another glass of wine, then took a sampling of the food. "This is terrific," she said in genuine admiration. "Why don't you open a Chinese restaurant? In the long run, I'm sure you'd be much happier."

He laughed. "I doubt it. You know, you're exaggerating. There is ample opportunity for developing, maybe not long lasting, but important relationships with the people who come in seeking help."

"I sure as heck didn't see it. I mean even when someone really sick comes in, what happens? Everyone runs to the patient, they do the workup, and take a thousand blood samples. Then someone looks at their watch and says, 'Heck, it's another forty minutes before the lab results will be back,' and everyone hurries over to the coffee machine to bullshit, leaving the patient flat on his back and counting the holes in the accoustical ceiling to forget he's scared. And you know what? I can see the reason for doing that. I mean, why get involved with a patient who, whether he goes home or is admitted into one of the wards, is going to be out of your life in a few minutes anyway?"

Allan went back to the stove and started on the second dish he had planned. "But you see, that's where—in regard to the trauma service, anyway—your judgment is incomplete," he said as he began a new ritual of mixing shrimp, sugar, sesame oil, snow peas, onions, soy sauce, and noodles in the wok "Our involvement with that patient who came in this afternoon didn't stop with his transfer to the recovery room. Until he wakes up and gives some signs of making it, we're going to have to deal with a distraught young woman who is convinced her husband is as good as dead and that she is going to have to raise two young children by herself."

"Oh, all right. So you'll go out there and hold her hand a couple of minutes while she's in the waiting room. Big deal."

"Now come on, Maggie. Giving a wife or a husband or a child support during those first few days is sometimes the toughest part of the job. And it doesn't get easier once the patient regains consciousness. In fact, it gets worse. If this guy does come out of it, it'll be months before he goes into physical therapy. In the meantime, somewhere in the back of her mind, his wife'll wonder from time to time if she might not have been better off if he had died. Suppose he never gets out of bed again, she asks herself in a moment of weakness. Suppose he is confined to a wheelchair the rest of his life. Suppose, she asks herself—and hates herself for doing so—suppose he can't ever get it up again."

They both ate in silence for a minute or two. Allan polished off the last of his shrimp and sat back, fully satisfied with his cooking and his meal.

"I saw your files before you came on the service and I know that psychiatry is your real interest. But Maggie, we need you for the next two months. You can really contribute, especially if your real desire is to work with patients. Work with the jogger's wife, work with him if he makes it. He's going to need a strong will to live, he'll need to be convinced that he can return to a productive life-style; they'll both have to be convinced that they still can have a meaningful relationship, that he can still be a good father. Help us out, Maggie. Don't write us off."

Maggie doodled with her chopsticks on her now-empty plate, then looked up. Her eyes were very large, very warm. "I'm sorry, I guess I was out of line. To tell you the truth, looking back on what happened, I was probably angrier at myself than at you."

"Why, because you couldn't do a cut-down in less than a minute your first time out?"

"Yes, in part. It's an old failing. I can't bear myself if I don't do something perfectly. I went through undergrad school and med school with only six B's and I'm convinced to this day they should have been A's as well. I just hate it when I screw up."

Allan started to clear the coffee table where they had eaten. "That's being pretty tough on yourself, isn't it? Demanding that you meet such rigorous standards."

"It's the way I grew up. The fact that I couldn't do the cut-down well enough to meet my standards was only a part of the reason for my blowing up."

"And the other part?"

"God, I know this is really going to sound Freudian, but the other part is that you remind me a lot of my father."

"Come on! What am I? Seven, eight years older than you?" They walked to the kitchen, each carrying a share of the plates that had accumulated in the course of the meal.

"It's not your age, it's the way you act," Maggie continued while scrounging under the sink and in assorted drawers for dishwashing supplies. "Before I came on the service I had seen you around the hospital. And I had certainly heard of you. You're known as the 'Trauma Terrorist.'"

Allan put down the towel with which he had been drying the dishes Maggie had been handing him. "Are you serious?"

Maggie looked at him skeptically. "You mean you'd never heard that before? Well, you might as well know. They say you go around issuing nonnegotiable demands that would make this a perfect world for trauma victims and if, God forbid, no one moves as fast as you want them to, you go into a terrorist routine that would do the Black September movement proud." She stopped, then laughed. "Look at you. I think you're actually enjoying this information."

Allan could feel himself flushing. "No, it's just that . . . Never mind. What's this have to do with your father?"

"He was like that. Impatient with an imperfect world.

Demanding that it and everyone in it live up to his exceedingly high standards of morality, professionalism, whatever."

Allan gathered up two cups, a jar of decaffeinated espresso, a kettle of hot water he had put on to boil, sugar and cream, placed it all on a tray and moved back to the living room couch. Maggie ignored the deep-cushioned chair she had favored while they were eating and sat down next to him. He sensed her body heat, a sensation that sent a tingling through his loins.

"And those high standards your father set for everyone included you, of course. Was he a physician?"

"Cardiologist. He had a huge following. Some foreign types, even finance ministers for little sheikhdoms in the Middle East, started coming all the way to the United States to consult with him when worrying about all those billions of petrodollars gave them too much angina. Definitely a star."

Maggie moved back toward one of the armrests, leaned against it, kicked off her shoes, and brought her legs up on the couch and folded them under her. Allan had not noticed it before, but her skin had an alabaster quality. Looking at it, at her black hair and her pitch-black eyes, he had a passing feeling that there was a very lifelike bust of a Greek goddess on his couch. For a moment Maggie caught and held his glance. She tilted her head a bit and smiled.

"Want me to go on?" It was a friendly question.

"Sorry. It's just that it just struck me that you are beautiful."

"Thank you. I'm glad you're noticing now, not the next time I try to do a cut-down. In any case, I worshipped my father. I wanted to be like him. I wanted to be him. He felt that it was his due as well, that I should carry on his tradition."

Maggie uncurled herself, poured herself another glass of wine. "And you?"

"And me what?"

"Why are you so driven? What's the secret behind your one-hundred-hour weeks, the research, the crazy demands on people that work for you—"

"They're not crazy demands. They're necessary. Damnit, Maggie. People's lives are at stake."

"Hip, hip, hoorah. Other people save lives too, Allan. But

they don't make their own lives and those of the people who work with them miserable in the process."

"So you think there's a Freudian secret behind me too?"

"Well?"

"I don't know that it's Freudian. But, yes, what you told me about yourself and your father sounds familiar."

Maggie said nothing.

"My father was a neurosurgeon. Chairman of the department at Emory. I have two sisters and a brother, but I was the only one who mattered to him. I was the one who was branded gifted at the age of seven. I was the one who got special tutoring in science and math. On Saturday and Sunday, my best friend's father coached his sandlot baseball and football teams and taught him how to hit or call plays. Mine took me to the hospital and taught me medicine. I don't know of any other fourteen-year-old who spent his Saturdays dissecting human brains or searching out the routes the major nerves take through the body."

"How awful!"

"That wasn't the awful part. It might even have been fun. What was awful was his rage when I couldn't differentiate between the pineal gland and the corpora quadrigemina or couldn't isolate the thalamus quickly enough. I would try and try and no matter how hard I tried, I couldn't please him."

"And of course he wanted you to be a neurosurgeon."

"Yes. He never understood why I would want to go into a mechanical subspecialty like trauma surgery. When I told him, he ranted and raved that he couldn't understand why I wanted to go into something that required no intellect. 'You are not to become the medical equivalent of an automobile mechanic,' is what he screamed."

"Boy. I really hit a sore spot when I spouted off this afternoon, didn't I?"

"That's the standard reaction. It doesn't bother me anymore. But anyway, he made growing up very hard for me."

The ensuing silence was broken by Maggie. "You know, Allan, I'm not so sure you really deserve that terrorist designation."

"Ah, well, just wait till I raise my arms and accidentally reveal the scalpel tucked close to my chest."

"No, seriously. These have been the best three or four hours I've spent in a long, long time. You know how to listen to someone."

Allan started to say something but Maggie leaned over and touched his mouth with her fingertips. Slowly she moved over and when she was very close to him, pulled her hand away, leaned toward him and kissed him. He felt himself respond. And yet, he was torn. It was Julie he was suddenly thinking about, Julie he wanted. But a voice inside him said don't be a fool. Julie hasn't given you the time of day. She's shut you off cold. As Maggie's hand caressed first the top of his thigh, then inside, thoughts of Julie evaporated. He felt himself relax completely and, though he had always made the first move with other women, this time he decided to follow Maggie's lead.

After they had disentangled, there was a silence. Allan felt awkward. He tried to guess what Maggie was thinking, but soon gave up.

"Listen," he said finally, when he saw that Maggie was not about to break the quiet.

"Shh," she said, still resting against him but not moving to look at him. "Don't go saying anything dumb you'll regret in the morning."

"But—"

"No buts. It happened. I loved the food. I loved you. I feel good. So shut up and relax. Don't get bent out of shape about what it all means. Okay?"

"Okay," Allan said, though not quite sure he sounded convincing.

"Good man. Now, are we going to spend the night on this couch, or do you own a decent bed?"

5

Allan had the receiver to his ear even before the clamoring of the first ring had fully died away.

"What?" he said, peering at the clock on the bed stand next to him. It was 4:10 A.M.

"It's our jogger," Santorre said. "His vital signs are starting to crap out. We've given him five more units of blood since you were here but despite that, his blood count still is falling. We're having trouble keeping his blood pressure above eighty systolic. His urine output has been negligible the last two hours."

"It sounds to me like we have to go back in. I'll be there in fifteen minutes."

Allan turned to wake Maggie but she was already up. "Bad?" she asked.

"Looks bad." He headed for the bathroom and Maggie followed.

They showered together to save time. Allan drew on pants, slipped into his loafers, and wrestled to pull on a sweatshirt as he walked into the kitchen. He flung open the refrigerator door and took out a jar of peanut butter, a jar of strawberry jam, and half a loaf of bread. Grabbing a knife from the dish rack where some of the plates and utensils from the previous evening's meal were drying, he ran to the front door, where Maggie was already waiting. "The young doctor's version of C-rations," he said, handing her the supplies. "Make us some sandwiches while I drive. It may be the only chance we'll have to eat all day."

"Yuck!" was Maggie's only response.

With Maggie at his heels, he strode past the four ambulances parked side by side at the emergency-room door, through the open doors, and, bypassing the elevator, up the stairs leading to the recovery room. Santorre had apparently been called away, because now David Fedder was standing next to the jogger's bed.

"Dave doesn't look much better than the patient," Maggie said, nodding toward Fedder, who was looking at the clipboard attached to the jogger's bed. The young man's greens were rumpled and wrinkled. His hair was at once matted and disheveled. His face looked puffy. There were formidable bags under his eyes.

"Where's Santorre?"

"Got called to the E.R. about another admit," Fedder answered. Despite his fatigue and his concern for the patient, he took note of Maggie's simultaneous appearance with Allan.

"Okay," Allan continued, ignoring the look Fedder had cast at them, "what have we got?"

"The guy is still bleeding on us. After Santorre called you he transfused two more units of fresh frozen plasma."

"Did it have any effect on his clotting studies?"

"It's confusing. His pro time and PTTs are almost normal, but his blood pressure continues to drop. He's on his seventh unit of blood since the operation, which makes a total of thirty-seven since he's come in."

"Which tells you what?" Allan, ever the teacher, asked.

"According to the lab, he should have the ability to clot, but I think he's still bleeding. If we don't do something to change the trend, we're going to lose him."

Allan moved toward the bed and Fedder stepped aside. Allan ran his fingers around the jogger's neck, down his chest, rested them lightly on his abdomen.

"What do you think?" It was Santorre, who had stepped back into the recovery room.

"His abdomen is obviously more distended and, yes, he is continuing to bleed. It has to be going into the abdomen. Let's go in."

"I'm ready," Fedder and Santorre said in unison.

Allan turned to Maggie, who had been standing silently off to the side. "See to it that we are ahead six units of whole blood. You're going to have to mobilize four units, minimum, of freshly drawn walking donor blood. The O.R. has the protocol to line up the necessary volunteer firemen and policemen. Just notify the front desk. Anybody around here A positive?"

"I am," Maggie volunteered. "I'll stop by the bank after I talk to the desk." Allan said a quiet "Thanks," then turned his attention back to the bed. Santorre, close to Allan's side, could not resist nudging him in the ribs.

The jogger, raw red bruises on his chest, his abdomen, and his flanks, a dribble of blood draining from the sutured incision spanning his chest and abdomen, was on the operating-room table, his bloodied bandages cut away and lying in a heap in a laundry cart. As nurses, residents, and interns jockeyed around each other in the crowded operating room, IV lines, drapes, instrument tables danced into position. The cardiac monitor above and to the left of the anesthesiologist blipped into action and began to draw the ragged electronic mountain ranges that traced the beats and rests of the jogger's heart.

Already scrubbed, Allan held out his hand and a nurse slapped scissors into it. Allan jabbed into the lower portion of the incision he had made during the first surgery on the man and quickly ran the instrument up toward the chest. The incision sprang open as if the jogger's skin were the peel of an overripe fruit strained by the accumulation of juices. Dark blood gushed out. Massive clots popped to the surface, revealing the jogger's innards.

Santorre cursed. "There's six to eight units of blood in here."

"You ever open up a belly when you haven't found more blood in there than you expected?" Allan asked, sweeping away the clots, then suctioning out the remaining blood. Starting on the left upper portion of the abdomen and working clockwise, he examined the jogger's insides inch by inch.

"It's in the back here, where we had all the bleeding around the pancreas," Allan finally said. "Lot of diffuse oozing going on. Hand me the electrocautery unit." Short bursts of buzzing from the cautery filled the operating room. The acrid smell of burning flesh crept through the air. Satisfied he had stemmed the bleeding in one spot, Allan moved to another, this time choosing to use sutures.

"It's coming from there too," Santorre said, pointing to a small trickle of blood coming from yet another part of the abdomen. Allan took a dozen quick stitches and the bleeding stopped in the spot Santorre had pointed out. But no sooner had Allan finished the chore than he noticed drops of blood in yet another area. A clearly discernible aura of desperation settled over the room as Allan, like a farmer desperately trying to patch a dike springing leaks anew from a dozen places, furiously shifted his attentions from oozing spot to oozing spot.

"It's no good," Allan finally said. "He's developing bleeding from new sites faster than we can control them. It has to be some kind of a clotting abnormality that's escaping us for the moment. How much of the fresh blood have we used?"

"Nearly all of it."

"Shit. If the fresh blood doesn't help him clot . . ." Allan didn't finish the sentence.

"He's going to crump on us," Fedder added, morosely.

"You're well on your way to being a surgeon, Fedder," Allan said. "A man is dying and you take it as a personal insult because he's cashing in on the O.R. table."

"You could try just packing him, get out, and hope that pressure helps those spots seal," Maggie said. She had finished donating blood and was now leaning over Allan's shoulder, watching him work.

"That's a little out of date, lady," Santorre said. "That was edited out of the textbooks when you were still playing nurse with your dolls."

Maggie, angered by the remark, started to reply but Allan cut in. "If we pack him, we run the risk of a rip-roaring infection a few days down the line. But right now an infection is the least of our worries because the packing could be our only chance to control the bleeding," Allan said. He mulled Maggie's suggestion over for a couple of seconds, then decided. "Okay, pack him and we'll come back in twenty-four or forty-eight hours. By then he should be replenishing his own clotting factors. It's risky, but it's our only shot."

The packing procedure finished, Allan and Santorre closed up. The team dispersed. Santorre and a nurse wheeled the jogger back to the recovery room. Fedder decided to return to the E.R.

"Think I'll practice some cut-downs on a cadaver or two until rounds," Maggie announced.

Allan stopped her. "That can wait, Maggie. His wife is still in the lounge. Spend some time with her. Talk to her for a while. Hold her hand. That's more important right now."

Hoping that the early morning air would dissolve some of the tension that had accumulated during the emergency surgery, Allan walked to his car to retrieve his stethoscope, then strolled slowly back to the emergency room. An ambulance had just arrived at the E.R. doors. The attendants were sliding a man out. His thin face was cadaverous, dry blood was crusted around his mouth. His large, sunken eyes were yellowish. There were no muscles on his naked arms and legs. His stomach was bulging, almost as if he were trying to sneak a basketball into the hospital beneath his dirty and torn shirt. He clawed and picked at the air, mumbling about the spiders attacking him. At first glance he seemed to be eighty years old, though Allan estimated his age was closer to forty.

One of the attendants noticed Allan passing. "Hey, doc," he yelled out, "look what we got for you."

Allan shook his head and said nothing. Another pumpkin, he thought to himself. Another alcoholic who, in all likelihood, was bleeding from ruptured veins in his esophagus. Night after night drunks like that were found in the flophouses of San Francisco and were rushed to the University hospital's emergency room. And night after night, twenty to thirty units of valuable blood would be pumped into the winos in the futile effort to save them.

Allan squeezed by the attendant and stepped back into the emergency room. The air, the seats, the floors were redolent with the traces left behind by the drunks, the hippies, the street people, the whores, the rough-trade gays, the ghetto and barrio residents, the cops, all the people who had paraded through in the last eight or ten hours seeking help for drug overdoses, miscarriages, knife wounds, bullet holes, tears in abused sexual organs, suicidal fits, ignored colds turned to incipient pneumonia, loneliness, and even hunger. The dayside janitorial crew had not yet cleaned, so the peculiar smell the previous night's patients had collectively left behind still lingered, that mixture of urine, feces, vomit, disinfectant, antiseptics, sweat and, from time to time, the surreptitiously smoked marijuana cigarette. Allan drew sustenance from the special aura the men, women, and children who passed through had created. Gathered together into one massive common denominator, they allowed medicine, time and again, to prove its ability to be of value to all of society.

The emergency room was nearly empty now. A young woman, cradling a small child, sat in one corner. A well-dressed man sat near her, casually leafing through a magazine. On the other side of the room, an elderly black man was sleeping, his legs stretched out in front of him, his head flopped back, his mouth open. Two policemen were leaning against the stained soft-drink machine, one reading softly aloud from a small notebook, the other sipping from a cup and listening.

Allan made his way to the nursing station and picked up the log book on the counter.

"Well! What's God's very own gift to trauma doing here? I thought this was the blue team's shift." It was the charge nurse, a sixty-two-year-old woman who still worked with the vigor of doctors and nurses thirty years younger. She had given in to the pleasant plumpness of a grandmother who bakes too much for her grandchildren.

"You're right, the blue team is on duty," Allan answered and pushed aside the book without bothering to read. "But a case we did yesterday afternoon turned sour. Anything exciting go on last night?"

"Didn't you watch the eleven-o'clock news?"

Allan, recalling with pleasure what he had been doing at eleven the previous night, shook his head.

"Cop was shot in the chest by a liquor-store burglar. He lucked out because it caught him on the right side and he got away with a hemopneumothorax and responded quickly to a chest tube. But all the television stations were here and the docs looked like heroes."

"Nice," Allan said, very much unimpressed.

"Fedder had a really hard night," she continued, obviously lobbying in the younger man's behalf. "Go easy on him."

"Putting in one chest tube and going on television for a round of public adulation doesn't sound too terribly hard to me."

"The cop wasn't all. We had another incident." She nodded to the two policemen by the soft-drink machine. "They're still trying to figure it out. But anyway. Fedder really worked his young you-know-what off on that one too."

Allan waited for the story.

"Three men were waiting at a bus stop down on Market where all that building is going on. One of them was about sixty-five, the other two in their twenties," the nurse continued. "All of a sudden, two of the men, one of the younger ones and the old man, just dropped to the ground, their legs cut out from under them."

"What do you mean, 'cut out from under them'?"

"Just that. One second they have legs, the next second the four legs are gone, cut off at mid-thigh. Without thinking, the third guy grabs the stumps of the young man and using his thumbs puts direct pressure on the spurting femoral arteries. Some cops who were in the area put a tourniquet on the older man.

"Fedder had a hell of a time because the older guy just wouldn't respond. He died about twenty minutes after he pulled in. The worst part was that Fedder couldn't pry the uninjured man's hands off the young guy's stumps. What we could get out of the third man was that the other young man was his brother. The older guy, the one who died, was their father. The kid really saved his brother's life, but he's a basket case because he feels so guilty about not being able to do anything about his father."

"Where is everybody now?"

"The man who lost his legs is up in the ICU. Fedder called up there about ten minutes ago. He's not out of the woods yet, but the guess is he's going to make it. We sedated the brother and the cops are waiting for him to wake up so they can question him and try to make some sense about what happened."

"And no one has any idea?"

"Nothing. One of the cops who came in with them last night said that someone else who had been waiting near the bus stop said it was like an invisible sword had cut through them. But that's all they could say. No one saw anything that would explain what happened."

Shaking his head, Allan walked toward the row of cubicles that served as treatment rooms. He passed one in which a young man was sleeping and three that were empty. He paused before the fifth one and drew aside the curtain that served as a privacy barrier. A young woman was lying on the table, an endotracheal tube protruding from her mouth. A single IV line was in her right arm. Fedder was on her left. Sandra Couzens, the physician who would be responsible for the emergency room for the day that was just beginning, was on the young woman's right. She was holding a stethoscope to the woman's chest, listening to breath sounds.

"What do you have?" Allan asked as he walked in.

"Nineteen-year-old kid who came home high on PCP," Couzens answered. "Opened her mother's medicine cabinet and swallowed everything in sight. Valium, Seconal, aspirin, Tylenol/codeine, diet pills, the lot."

"How's she doing now?"

Fedder answered. "She's coming around, starting to breathe on her own. They got her in here pretty fast, so that helped. You going to make rounds with us?"

"Yeah, I have some time, but I can't take too long. I have a meeting with Phil Dorr in about an hour. Anything in the minor trauma room we should look at?"

"Nah. The one interesting case is gone. Young heroin addict came in. He had run out of veins to inject so for the last month he's been shooting up in the dorsal vein of his prick. He told me he thought he had a hernia but when he dropped trou what he showed me was one hugely gangrenous cock. I told him he should be admitted but he refused, even when I told him we'd put him on methadone so he wouldn't go into withdrawal while he was here. He signed out against medical advice. Other than that, the usual assortment of abscesses to be drained, lacerations sutured. Crap."

"Female trauma room?" Couzens asked. The short questions were the hallmark of the woman, who had decided to become a doctor after ten years as a medical technician. She was short, plump. Her hair was closely cropped and she stared out at the world through small brown eyes made smaller by the owlish wire-rim glasses she favored. She seldom smiled, never socialized with the other emergency-room or trauma-service doctors. Allan had once speculated on what her life away from the hospital was like. He came to the conclusion that she did not exist away from the hospital. He decided that when it came time for her to be on duty she materialized outside the E.R. doors; when her shift was over, she stepped outside and simply evaporated.

"Two spontaneous abortions, a case of gonorrhea, two hysterics who made suicide gestures," Fedder recounted. "That's about it."

They reached the male admitting ward. Allan stepped up to a small narrow door and tried it. When he realized it was locked, he peered into the room through a window laced with wire mesh. Against a distant corner, curled into a small human ball, lay a nude man. He didn't move.

"What's his story?" Allan asked.

"Cops brought him in. He was standing, *au naturel*, on one of the pedestrian walkways at the Embarcadero, screaming he was Julius Caesar, that Christ had sent him to save the world. Took five cops to get him under control and then hold him down here while we got some Thorazine into him. We've been trying to find a bed for him, but no luck so far."

They came to a bed holding an unconscious man of about fifty. "He was found like that over in the Nob Hill area, lying in the street," Fedder said. "No evidence of trauma. The internists think he had an intracerebral hemorrhage."

Couzens took a small reflex hammer from her back pocket and banged on the man's Achilles tendon. Nothing moved. Taking a needle she jabbed him in various spots on his arms and legs. Again, no response.

"We already know he's unresponsive to painful stimuli, Couzens," Allan said, annoyed.

"No harm checking."

"When are they going to admit him?" Allan asked.

"He should have been up there an hour ago. But you know the internists. God forbid anything should interfere with breakfast. They'll get around to claiming him when they're done with their second cup of coffee, I guess," Fedder answered. "I've still got surgery clinics. Do me a favor, will you, Couzens? Clean all this crap out of here by the time I get back."

Allan took his leave as well and, bounding up a staircase, went to the ICU. Santorre was at the jogger's bedside, writing on a clipboard.

"What's happening?" Allan asked.

"Nothing much, which is good, I guess. His vitals are stable. His pulse rate is coming down. No bleeding from the incision. His blood count is stable, so maybe Maggie's packing is starting to do the trick." Santorre looked up from the clipboard. "I guess I'll have to make nice to her later."

"I'd say that would be appropriate. Can you give me a quick rundown on our patients here?"

"Okay. The cop who was shot in the chest is stable and I think we can get him out of here and onto the floor today. The kid who fell off his skateboard and hit his head against the curb, we should have him off the respirator this afternoon and I think we can give him to pediatrics tomorrow. The guy who took on the Muni bus is still on a ventilator. He'll need a tracheostomy in the next day or two."

"What about the kid whose legs were cut off in that . . . well, in whatever it was that happened?"

"He seems to be holding his own. I think he'll make it."

"I forgot to ask downstairs. Whatever happened to his legs?"

"The cops did bring them in, even managed to package them in ice. But he was just not in any kind of shape for us to consider reattaching them. He's twenty-two and it'll be tough for him to adjust to the amputation, but it's the best he could have hoped for."

"Have you heard anything more on what caused it?"

"Yeah, I just talked to the cops a couple of minutes ago. Christ, talk about bizarre. There's a building going up across the street from where those guys were waiting for the bus. The cable in an elevator shaft snapped and the damned thing went spinning off at a high velocity. It came at them, sliced them up and just kept going down an alley behind them. They found the cable two blocks away."

Phil Dorr, the hospital's chief of staff and Allan's mentor and spiritual adviser, smiled broadly when Allan strode into his office. Dorr was a handsome sixty-year-old man who, despite a thick mane of gray hair, looked ten years younger. Rosy cheeks—according to him, the result of huffing and puffing on an exercise bicycle for half an hour every day—accented an open, relaxed face. They shook hands, Dorr taking the opportunity, as always, to slap Allan on the back. But the instant Allan sat down in one of the straight-back oak chairs in front of Dorr's desk, the older man walked back to the massive executive chair behind his desk and turned serious. His hands, forming a steeple, lightly touched his lips. He regarded Allan intently.

"You proud of yourself, Allan?"

Allan, uncomfortable because he recognized Dorr's approach to an unpleasant subject, squirmed in his seat. "Proud?" he echoed in what he knew was a dumb attempt to stall for time.

Dorr lapsed into silence, continuing to stare directly at Allan.

"Really. I don't know what you're talking about. Or not talking about. Or whatever." Allan was well aware that he was babbling.

"Allan, you know how important you are to this institution, don't you? You know the value of your work. Or at least I hope you do."

Now Allan knew for certain a lecture was coming.

"Allan. How can you possibly take two units of whole blood, walk into the administrator's office, who we all know hates the sight of it, and just simply pour it over his desk like that? Don't you have any sense . . ."

The reminder of his confrontation with Jack White rallied

Allan. "Oh, come on, Phil. Don't talk down to me. In the first place, I didn't pour them over his desk. I slapped them down and the bags split open. In the second place, yes, I know better. But goddamnit, we've been pleading for a portable blood cooler for the trauma O.R. for months. We waste more blood. . . ."

"I'm not disputing the need, Allan," Dorr's voice had lost a little bit of its warmth. "Just your methods."

"My methods? I asked, I pleaded, I wrote memos, I sent copies of articles about blood conservation from *Circulation*. I had six different hospital-supply houses send brochures and walked two salesmen up to his office personally. Nothing helped, Phil. And a blood cooler is no minor matter."

"I grant you that. But the man is powerful and now you have managed to alienate him beyond redemption." He stopped and again aimed a concentrated stare at Allan. "And a man in your position is going to need as many friends as possible."

Allan, who had been slouching in his chair, bolted upright. "Has the appointment gone through?"

"It has in a sense, yes. Yesterday afternoon, the board of directors finally approved our plan to create a separate section for trauma in the surgical division."

Allan leaped out of his chair. "That's terrific!"

"Yes, it is. The point, though, is that the board is going to be scrutinizing the section very carefully. There was a lot of antagonism about creating it, a lot of worrying that it would drain off resources needed elsewhere. Cardiac surgery has been lobbying for another O.R. and new heart-and-lung machine and they argued that a hell of a lot more people have heart attacks than trauma problems. Cancer wanted to expand the interferon and the monoclonal-antibody program and were not supportive. And, most of all, nobody was terribly eager to make you head of a department."

"But you sold them."

"Yes. And they sort of bought you. They wouldn't go for a hard-and-fast appointment, but approved you only as temporary head. A good thing we met before the story of the blood got out." Dorr stood up, walked around to the front of the desk, and sat down on one corner. He looked down at Allan. "If that trauma section is going to survive and if you want the appointment as its permanent head, you are going to have to grow up."

"You mean play the political game," Allan flared.

"Call it whatever you want. You managed to get your trauma teams going because you have an undeniable ability for leadership and because you are a first-rate surgeon. You're enthusiastic about trauma and you work hard at it—too hard, I sometimes think. But those are the qualities that have residents and interns around here competing to work with you. And there's no denying you're pulling off miracles."

"So why do I have—"

"—to practice a little political acumen? Because even though there's a lot of admiration around here for what you've done, there is also a lot of latent resentment. You're competing for limited resources and that means that, whether you like it or not, you're going to have to start building relationships with some of the people around here who matter."

"If you want me to start kissing ass . . ."

"You don't have to kiss ass, Allan. Look, for the last twenty years the center's 'Golden Apple for Teaching Excellence' has gone to an outstanding teacher, to someone on the faculty."

"I won it this year."

"Exactly my point. The award is voted by the students, it always has gone to a medical type. You were the first surgeon to be honored that way. Why?"

"Because—"

"Yes, I know. Because you deserved it."

"Not just that I deserved it, but if you want me to be honest, because I'm dedicated and because I'm uncompromising in teaching and, more important, I'm uncompromising when it comes to treating patients. The residents, interns, and medical students appreciate that."

"There you go. That's exactly the problem with you, Allan. You think you are the only one in this institution who has any scruples, the only one who cares about patients or students. But even if that were true, let's be honest. That award is something of a popularity contest as well. You know as well as I that it could have gone to any one of a dozen people. The students voted it to you because they love you. They worship you."

"I don't know that they worship me. They respect me and what I'm trying to do."

"They respect a lot of people. The difference is that you treat them like human beings."

"I can be pretty rough on the people who work with me too. Ask Maggie Brooks."

"I'm sure you verbally keelhaul them too from time to time. But it's a different kind of harshness. It's one that's forgotten because—and I've seen you do it—it is often followed by some friendly gesture, a word of encouragement, or by an effort on your part to make sure that some medical lesson was learned. All I'm getting at is that you can start treating some of your ranking colleagues the same way. It won't cost you much. And if you don't, believe me, it'll cost you dearly and nothing I can do will save you. Will you give it a try?"

Allan nodded. "Sure."

"Now, tell me. How's your work with the artificial blood going?"

Allan froze. Was it possible that Dorr had heard about what had happened at Coit Hill, that he had tried, without authorization, to use some of his experimental artificial blood in a last-ditch effort to save the biker? Who could possibly have found out?

To his profound relief, there was a light tapping on the door. The chief of staff's secretary thrust her head into the room.

"Sorry to disturb you, but I thought it might be important," she said. "Dr. Kirk, a Miss McDonough at the medical examiner's office asks you call her when you have a chance."

"Allan, the artificial blood?" Dorr said, laughing. Allan realized that on hearing Julie's name, he had momentarily tuned everything else out.

"Sorry. I was just trying to remember what I had filled you in on and what I hadn't. Have I told you that an NIH team is coming out in a couple of weeks to look at what we're doing?"

"No, you have not been very communicative about that part of your life."

"Sorry. Anyway, I've been setting up a demonstration experiment for a National Institutes of Health team that is coming out to survey us." Allan glanced at his watch. "Give me about an hour so I can get a dog ready, then come over to the lab and I'll preview my spiel for you."

Allan asked one of his laboratory technicians to prepare a dog for his session with Dorr, then let himself into his small office. As he dialed, he castigated himself for feeling butterflies flit about his stomach, flitting that increased when Julie answered the phone.

"I just wanted to let you know that I found about half a dozen cases for you among some of the files that haven't gone on the shelf yet," she said after they had exchanged hellos.

"Thanks. I appreciate that. But you don't have to. . . ."

"I had the time. The cases were handy."

He was sure there was a hidden purpose to her call, that she probably felt bad about the chilly way in which she had rebuffed him after their return from the fair in Santa Rosa. A desire to help her achieve a thaw in their personal relationship battled with an unwillingness to suffer another curt dismissal like the one he had been subjected to in the medical examiner's parking lot. His determination to keep matters on a professional basis won out, though he felt none too happy about the victory.

"I should be by there in a few days and I can pick them up," he said. "Or just put them in the mail for me."

"All right," she said, her voice dropping a bit. "Give me your address."

Upset and confused, Allan returned to his laboratory. A dog of German shepherd ancestry lay on one of the operating tables. A tube ran from the animal's windpipe to a ventilator. Because the tube pushed back the upper portion of the dog's mouth and in the process retracted the animal's upper lip, the animal seemed to be smiling in his sleep, satisfied that he was giving his life up for the sake of mankind. Allan washed up and helped the technician open the animal's chest and belly, place tubes in various blood vessels, and connect sensors to key muscles and organs.

"Ready?" asked Dorr, who had slipped into the laboratory as Allan and the technician were making their final preparations.

"Sure!" Allan responded with enthusiasm. "You want me to give you the whole pitch?"

"Might as well."

"Okay." Allan turned to the operating table and turned valves on several of the transparent tubes sprouting from the dog. Blood began to flow through them to the reservoir tank hidden beneath the table. The technician flipped switches on equipment standing near the table and the soft whirring of electrical motors filtered through the air. Light green digital numbers flicked back and forth on three small boxes.

Allan took a deep breath. "The whole speech, including the basics?"

"Might as well. Let's critique that as well."

"Okay. Shock, the damage caused the body by the steady and unchecked loss of blood, is the single greatest threat facing the trauma patient immediately after he has been injured. By and large, if we want to save a seriously traumatized patient we have an hour—the so-called Golden Hour—in which to do so. If we let any more time than that go by, shock becomes irreversible."

"You might want to say something about the effects of shock on the various parts of the body, don't you think?"

"Yes. That is why the dog." Allan thought for a second. "By now the animal has lost about a third of its blood volume, and yet, like the trauma victim out in the field, he looks deceptively stable. His pulse rate is near normal. His blood pressure readings are stable.

"But as blood loss continues, we see subtle changes coming about. You can see that the heart's contractions are harder because the organ is working harder to maintain the same amount of oxygen tension in the tissues as if the blood flow were normal. Let's wait a few minutes now and wait to see what happens as the dog continues to lose blood."

Dorr, folding his arms across his chest, leaned against the second operating table in the laboratory. Allan fixed his gaze on the filling reservoir, watching as its red liquid inched up. The technician brought two long racks to the table, each holding two filled containers, then ran intravenous lines from the containers to two veins in the dog's legs.

"The dog has now lost half of its blood volume and you can see that blood pressure is falling," Allan continued. "There are alterations in the brain-wave readings. There is evidence of severe muscle acidosis. If we let the situation go unchecked, we could expect that the dog would suffer cardiac arrest within another ten minutes or so."

Allan walked to the IV lines the technician had set up and started the flow of the liquids in the containers. "This artificial blood we have been working on here," he continued, "is designed to do more than just match the volume of blood escaping through an injury. It is meant to carry oxygen to all parts of the body, thus minimizing, if not eliminating, the major cause of shock, oxygen starvation."

He motioned to Dorr. "Come on, I'll show you." They walked to one of the machines attached with wires to the dog's body. As they watched, the soft-green digital numbers on the machine's window began to change, the values growing larger and larger.

"The effect," Allan said, "is virtually immediate. But let me tell you this. In this animal, because we waited so long to give him the artificial blood, it won't have all the impact it could."

"Let me go on role playing here, Allan," Dorr interrupted. "Why would it have a limited impact?"

"Because, for the sake of the demonstration, I've allowed the shock process to go too far and it has taken much of its toll. At so late a point, you might help the patient buy some time, perhaps enough to buffer him against any temporary delays in getting him to the operating room, but not a heck of a lot beyond that."

"Then why bother pursuing this at all?"

"Because what we have found in our research is that if you infuse a dog early in the bleeding process, within the first ten or fifteen minutes, you gain at least two, sometimes three, hours before the animal begins to suffer from the shock damage that is likely to kill him. In other words, if this artificial blood were to be given to a patient in the field by the paramedics, that Golden Hour in which he must have surgery to control his bleeding would be stretched into two, if not three, Golden Hours. It's in the field that we want to begin using it."

"Very impressive. But what are the obstacles?"

"Some of the early versions—not ours—of artificial blood relied on artificial molecules the developers hoped would behave like real blood. That is, the molecules that made up the product were designed to pick up oxygen in areas where there were high concentrations of oxygen—the lungs, of course—and then let go of the oxygen where concentrations were low—in the tissues around the body. But some of these early products were awfully good at latching onto the oxygen but weren't too good at letting go of it. And there were other problems. In the beginning, the molecules used to make artificial blood were too small. They just filtered out of the body through the kidneys, oxygen load and all.

"The army is experimenting with artificial blood made of real blood components. What they have done is take hemoglobin to transport oxygen from red blood cells, process the hemoglobin, purify it, and then use it in experimental work. Their approach is interesting but it also has not solved everything.

"We have been trying to work with a fluorocarbon molecule that will combine with oxygen in areas of high concentrations like the lungs and give off the oxygen in places where there is low concentration, like the tissues around the body. And, we have recently modified the molecule so that it does not simply pour through the kidney as if the molecule were going through a sieve."

"And?"

"And we have tested it on laboratory animals. The solution we just used on this dog is made up of our new formula. You saw the results. Oxygenation in the various tissues was up quickly after we administered it. But there are still questions we have to answer. What is the long-term toxic effect on humans? Will it damage the liver, the kidneys? How will it be metabolized? Will it lower a patient's ability to fight off disease? To answer those questions we want permission to begin clinical trials."

Dorr applauded politely. "Not bad. But I think you also need to remind your visitors that the artificial blood would be useful because, among other things, it would be free of diseases like hepatitis, AIDS, syphilis, which all occur in regular blood transfusions. Better yet, you will never have to worry about identifying blood types. Okay?"

"Sure. No harm in a little hard sell."

Allan and Dorr walked slowly out of the laboratory. As they approached Dorr's office, an older man—Allan judged him to be in his mid-fifties—who had been sitting in a lone chair near the office door, jumped up to greet them. He was thin, though the rumpled vest of his three-piece suit could not hide the markings of a potbelly. He was bald, and dark rim glasses accented a somber expression. He introduced himself as Sam Younger, the medical writer for the San Francisco *Telegraph*.

"If you want an interview, you'll have to go through the center's public information office," Dorr said. "They arrange all these sort of things."

Younger looked annoyed. "If you don't mind, I'm here already. I'm working on a story involving trauma and—"

Dorr smiled broadly. "Well, if you want to talk trauma, we can bypass the public information office for once. Especially since it's not my time you'll be taking up." Dorr bowed to Allan. "Doctor, this is your show. Handle it well." And with a wink, Dorr disappeared into his office.

"Why is this your show?" Younger asked.

"That's Dr. Dorr's idea of making a formal announcement about an appointment. I'm going to be temporary head of the new trauma surgery section the University is setting up. I'm Allan Kirk. Simple name to spell."

They ambled down the corridor. Younger was well informed about trauma and they talked easily about the new department. Allan, feeling as proud as the fathers they passed as they walked by the hospital's maternity center, chatted about the trauma team and the goals they hoped to achieve.

"You going to buy yourself a helicopter?" Younger asked, taking, for the first time, a small black mini tape recorder from his pocket.

"What the hell do I need a helicopter for? This isn't Vietnam."

"I just saw a study that showed that using helicopters to transport trauma victims could increase their chances of survival by better than fifty percent. In any case, Coit Hill has one, so why are you so disdainful of them?"

"First of all, Coit Hill has a lot of shiny, but useless, hardware. Second, I read the same study. And if I remember correctly, the study emphasized that the greatest benefit was to patients who had been hurt in remote areas where they were a long way from a trauma center. You don't need a helicopter in an urban setting."

Younger peered anxiously at his little recorder to make sure it was working. "Damned things," he apologized. "But a hell of a lot better than trying to write notes. Anyway. We heard that there was a flap over a patient the Coit Hill helicopter was supposed to pick up yesterday afternoon."

Allan stopped dead in his tracks. "A flap? What do you mean?"

"Jogger trying to cross Marina Boulevard was hit by a hit-and-run car yesterday."

"An ambulance brought him here. So?"

"That may be. But the guy was supposed to go to Coit Hill. The radio base station at Coit Hill told the paramedics to support the guy on the scene until their helicopter got there. When the chopper got there all they found was a bunch of people playing volleyball. Al Anthony was a might pissed that the paramedics had disregarded the hospital's instructions."

"Well, too bad. Sometimes paramedics misunderstand. . . ."

"It doesn't seem to be a case of misunderstanding. Apparently one of the paramedics, Drake his name is, just disconnected the base station because he didn't think it appropriate to take the jogger to Coit Hill."

Allan struggled to keep a poker face.

"In any case, the other paramedic squealed and Anthony, the administrator over there, went on the warpath. He pushed enough buttons to have Drake fired."

"Anthony had the paramedic fired?"

"Summarily."

"That stupid, power-hungry son of a bitch!"

"Why do you say that? The medic was wrong, wasn't he? Even if what you say about the study is right, the fact remains that in the helicopter that jogger would have been at Coit Hill five or six minutes sooner. And those minutes could be crucial, isn't that right?"

Allan walked away from the reporter. He shoved his hands deep into the pockets of the starched white laboratory coat he had put on after running through his demonstration for Dorr. His stomach was churning and he felt almost light-headed as the anger began to take hold of him. He wheeled back to face Younger.

"Of course he might have gotten to Coit Hill five minutes faster. So what? Would they have had a surgeon waiting? An anesthesiologist? A full set of operating-room nurses? Would they have had a bypass machine ready in case there was cardiac damage?"

He was out of control now. "Where does that jerk get off having someone fired? The paramedic should get a medal, goddamnit. Everybody in emergency knows Coit Hill's E.R. can't get surgical help in when the chips are down. Helicopter. What the hell good is a helicopter if you haven't got a commitment from your staff to back up the E.R.? Jesus, doesn't anybody understand what Anthony is doing? He's got a grandiose administrative scheme to set up some kind of a trauma service but he just doesn't have the support of his surgeons. He's putting together an empty shell!"

Younger, his hand holding the tape recorder at waist level, took a few steps toward Allan. "What you are saying is that Coit Hill endangers people in its emergency room?"

Allan's gaze fell on the little machine and rationality washed back over him.

"I wasn't saying anything of the sort, I was just asking some questions."

Younger pressed on. "You said that people who are in this field know the Coit Hill E.R. can't get help."

Allan, aware he was in trouble, tried to backpedal. "The truth is, no one can. Community hospitals generally have a hard time bringing in consultants at odd hours. It's a widespread problem."

"So what you're saying is that no hospital in San Francisco is capable of handling trauma cases but yours."

"Well, you can draw your own conclusions. I've said too

much already." And with that, Allan brushed past the reporter. Younger pressed first one button on his tape recorder, then another, and held it up to his ear. Satisfied that it had captured their conversation, he shut it off, took the small cassette out, carefully put it in a vest pocket, and began to look for the corridor that would take him out of the hospital.

6

He had spent twenty minutes driving up and down California, Sacramento, and Clay looking for a parking place. What a city, he muttered to himself. They put in a Residents Only parking plan, you have to screw around getting a sticker for your car and you still can't find a parking place when you come home at night. With a vehement "Screw it!" he pulled into a red space near a fire hydrant, locked the doors, and walked back to the small duplex where he lived.

Approaching the building, Allan could see a figure in the dark, outlined against the steps. Because San Francisco's street people wandered even into this, a supposedly better neighborhood, he approached with little concern, though when the figure rose and walked toward him with more than a hint of determination, he could feel his heart rate pick up. That the figure turned out to be Julie did nothing to calm him. He slowed, stopped, and waited for her to reach him.

"Now that you're sure I'm not a murderer," she said after a moment, "can we go in?" Puzzled, he said nothing. She turned and led the way. His watch told him it was almost midnight.

When he had opened the door and turned on the stair light,

she handed him a folded newspaper. "Well, Mr. Medical Macho, you've gone and done it, haven't you?" She swept by him and marched up the stairs. Allan, disturbed by her remark, stumbled after her, walked into the living room, and turned on light after light.

"I don't understand it, Allan," she said, stationing herself next to the couch, her arms folded across her chest. "You said your first stop was not going to be at the newspapers." Julie took off her windbreaker. Beneath it she was wearing a loose T-shirt that ended just above her navel and gray, baggy warm-up pants that sat comfortably at the top of her hips, just below her taut and narrow waist.

After an almost furtive look at the small, but enticing, trace of firm flesh that peeked out at him from between Julie's shirt and pants, Allan opened the newspaper and scanned its front page. He desperately tried to understand her caustic remarks. Only when his gaze fell on a box in the lower left-hand corner did he understand.

"'University Trauma Expert Slams Coit Hill Copter, Community Hospital E.R.'s,'" he read out loud. "Oh, shit!"

"Wait till you read the rest of it."

He ignored her and continued reading:

A $500,000 helicopter used by Coit Hill Memorial Medical Center to transport critically injured accident victims is a shiny piece of equipment that adds little of substance to patient care, a University trauma expert said today.

When Coit Hill officials launched their helicopter service they cited the role these aircraft played in the evacuation and treatment of soldiers in Vietnam and said their craft would prove to be a significant factor in helping save the lives of automobile or industrial accident victims.

But, according to Dr. Allan Kirk, acting head of the University of San Francisco's new Trauma Surgery Section, the advantage gained through a quick helicopter ride is lost because often surgeons are not available at Coit Hill when the craft arrives with a patient.

Coit Hill often cannot provide the services needed to save

patients who need immediate surgical care if they are to survive, Kirk said.

As a result, the use of a helicopter at Coit Hill, Kirk charged, represents only "a grandiose administrative scheme."

Coit Hill, Kirk said, is not the only hospital in San Francisco unable to cope with badly injured accident victims. Virtually every hospital, he said, has difficulties "bringing in consultants [specialists like surgeons] at odd hours. It's a widespread problem."

Studies in other parts of the nation, including Illinois, Maryland, Orange County, and Los Angeles, have consistently yielded data showing that up to 50 percent of trauma deaths occur because accident victims are treated in emergency rooms staffed by physicians who have not been trained to resuscitate the trauma patient or meet his complex needs or because surgeons do not respond in a timely manner.

Though a similar study has not been conducted in the San Francisco area, Kirk's contention that Bay area hospitals cannot muster medical help for trauma patients implies that a high percentage of them may be dying needlessly as well. . . .

Julie walked over to him and snatched the paper out of his hands. "You still haven't answered my question," she said. "Why did you go to the media?"

Allan sank into the couch. Dorr would be upset. Jack White, the University administrator, who was so proud of the good relations he managed to maintain with the other hospitals, would have a fit. The medical community would be outraged.

"Allan!"

He was startled out of his reverie. "I didn't go to the media," he said softly. "Younger came to us. He wanted to talk to Dorr, our chief of staff, but Dorr dumped him on me. I thought he wanted to do a story about our trauma work." He filled her in quickly on Anthony's move against the paramedic, on the rage he had felt at hearing of the firing.

Seeing Allan's mortification, Julie softened somewhat. Coming over to him, she gently put her hand on his shoulder. "Damn you, Allan. You are going to have to learn some self-control." Her voice was soft. "What do you think the fallout is going to be?"

Her touch calmed him down. "I have no idea. I'll probably get a pretty good dressing-down tomorrow. I'm going to be on a lot of shit lists for a long time."

"Well, you'll be lucky if that's all." She walked to the coffee table and sat on it.

Alarm spread over Allan's face. "What do you mean?"

"You *are* a babe in the woods! In the first place, medical people don't take too kindly to criticism, especially public criticism from someone in their own ranks. Unless I'm very wrong, you're in for not just a dressing-down or two, but a pretty good censure from the county medical association. Allan, you must know that until two years ago, any doctor who wanted to talk to the press, even about nice things, first had to get official clearance from the association's communications committee.

"Beyond that, if you had bothered to read something besides your medical journals, you'd know that Younger has been writing about emergency rooms for six months now. Every opportunity he gets he points out that there are delays in the care patients get in emergency rooms, that emergency rooms are more interested in a patient's ability to pay than in his medical needs, and that they unceremoniously dump patients who can't pay on county facilities. He's never had anyone talk about the problems on the record. And now suddenly there you come along, spouting off."

At a loss for an answer, Allan leaned back on the couch and rubbed his eyes with the heels of his hands. He just stared at her sitting there before him, one foot on the floor, the other resting on her knee. It suddenly dawned on him that in the flurry of excitement, he had not wondered at Julie's appearance on his doorstep in the middle of the night.

"In any case," he said, trying to be matter of fact. "Thanks for bringing it over." By now he knew better than to ask her directly about her actions.

"It's okay. I felt like getting out of the house. I went for a walk. I picked up the evening edition of tomorrow's paper on the way."

Silence seeped back into the room. Allan thought back to the first time he saw Julie, that morning at the medical examiner's office. In the first meeting she had been warm, friendly in a completely unguarded way. Yet until this moment, she had never been that open, that relaxed again. As he studied her now, she made no effort to withdraw.

Slowly, he sat forward. He put his hand under her chin and gently drew her toward him. Though she made no overt response, she did not resist either. He put his lips to hers, first just touching them, then kissing her gently, finally forcing her mouth open. Excited, yet also apprehensive that at any moment she would free herself from his embrace and flee, he put his hands on her shoulders, lifted her off the table, and guided her to the couch next to him. She followed. He drew back and looked at her. Her face was impassive.

He caressed her right cheek, passed his hand to the back of her head, and brought her to him again. He felt the touch of a hand on his shoulder, and chose to interpret it as encouragement. Barely breathing, he ran his hand down to her shoulder, lightly down her arm, and then across to her breast. Though she was putting a bit more passion into her kiss and though she was now gripping his shoulder, she was still somehow remote. Carefully, he lowered his hand to the bottom of her T-shirt, put his hand inside and moved it to the narrow cleavage between her breasts so that he could softly caress both at the same time. Almost imperceptibly she moved toward him.

He lowered his head and kissed the outline her breasts made against the T-shirt. Julie raised her arms and Allan helped her out of the garment. He kissed the side of her neck, her throat, the top of her chest. Slowly, relishing the opportunity, fearing it would suddenly disappear or never come again, Allan covered her breasts with soft kisses. When he felt her hesitatingly respond, he took one nipple in his mouth, slowly passing his tongue over it.

His qualms left him. He caressed the small of her back, slid his hand inside the top of her panties and ran it back and forth across the top of her buttocks, then across her hip and to the front until he could feel the downy texture of her hair. Her hands were resting on his back now, but an increase in the pressure of her fingertips was her only response. She put her head into the crook between his shoulder and his neck, rubbing her forehead back and forth against him. He kissed the top of her head, her temple, nudged her head up so that he could kiss her mouth. He withdrew his hand and, taking hold of the top of her pants, pulled them down, at the same time pushing Julie back on the couch. Her eyes were closed. His excitement growing quickly, he stepped out of his pants, straddled her, and lowered himself, working himself into position to enter her. He exhaled slowly in pleasure as he felt the tip of his hard flesh begin to sink into her.

"Jim," she cried out. "Jim. Oh, God, Jim. Please!"

Wildly, Allan jumped up and looked behind him, for a second convinced that someone else was in the apartment. Julie drew up her knees and rolled on her side. She was sobbing now, her head buried in her arms.

Allan sat on the edge of the couch, taking deep breaths, trying to calm his wildly beating heart. "Who in God's name is Jim?" His voice was hoarse.

Julie, crying quietly, said nothing. He got up, put on his pants, and walked to the kitchen for a glass of water. When he returned, Julie was dressed, sitting on the couch. He had no idea what to say.

"Do you have some wine?" she asked.

Allan nodded and went into the kitchen. He came back carrying a full glass and the bottle of wine. Julie emerged from the bathroom. She had washed her face and combed her hair. Her eyes were bloodshot and she was pale. He gave her the glass. She accepted it without a word and took a long draught. Then she sat down on the couch and leaned back, avoiding meeting his eyes.

"Would you mind telling me what that was all about? Who is Jim?"

She took another sip. Then a third one. Her voice was low. "The man I was going to marry."

She lowered her head. Allan, though afraid now to upset her, couldn't stay away. He sat next to her on the couch. "What do you mean, *was*?" Allan asked.

"The week after I got my master's, my family gave me a graduation party. Actually, it was more than that. I had been seeing Jim for three years and we had decided to get married. So it was going to be an engagement party too. It was a beautiful party. My aunt had rented out a restaurant on the dock at Tiburon and she invited about two hundred people for dinner. My family. His family. The works. It went on till one in the morning. Jim and I were the last ones to leave.

"He had an apartment here in the city so we decided to drive back to his place. But we were really high and feeling good, and Jim suggested we drive up to Twin Peaks. We drove up there and parked. We sat there for an hour just watching the lights of the city.

"There's kind of a low wall up there. There was no one around. We made love. Out in the open. Above the city." Julie started to cry again, but took a deep breath and stopped herself.

"About three or so, we started down. I don't know how it happened, but the car went out of control on a sharp curve. We must have crashed near a house because when I regained consciousness there were cop cars and ambulances everywhere. They took us to a hospital. But Jim died there before morning."

As Julie refilled her glass, Allan stood by, trying to think of something to say beyond the conventional "I'm sorry." It was the stock phrase he used when he talked to relatives of people who had died and now it seemed even more foolish and inadequate. Trying to end the awkward silence, he settled for "And you?"

"I was a basket case for a year. Didn't work, didn't go out. Finally, I decided I had to go on living so I started looking for work. The first job that came up was at the M.E.'s office. They were looking for a statistician and they hired me. I struggled with myself for months. I knew I shouldn't do it. But in the end, I did. I found the postmortem on Jim. The M.E. had decided that he bled to death of a liver laceration." Her voice broke. "A goddamn liver laceration that could have been controlled with a few sutures." She paused to take a deep breath.

"Anyway. After that I started the calls. It was going to be my way of getting people at the hospitals to pay more attention to the real causes behind the deaths of trauma victims."

Or maybe, Allan thought as he watched her take the last sip from the glass, your way of doing penance for having survived.

Gloria Cluny sat on the edge of the chair, her back straight, her hands, clasped, resting on her knees. Anthony, the morning paper lying open on his desk, took another sip of coffee from his mug. "Go on," he said after she had finished introducing herself and reminding him of her position on the staff.

"When I saw the paper this morning, Mr. Anthony, I was beside myself. The nerve of that man! To criticize us in that fashion . . ."

"Very unprofessional, I agree," Anthony said, wondering why she was taking up his time, but careful to be polite to her. "Especially when he has worked for us himself."

"Precisely! Why, you should have seen him carry on the night a young college boy died here, Mr. Anthony. Dr. Kirk went crazy when they brought that young boy in. He started ordering us all around as if we were first-year nursing students. He was highly offensive to the doctors who were on call. Why, you should have heard the language and the tone of voice he used with them, especially Dr. Harper. As if he were talking to plumbers who didn't want to come out in the middle of the night to fix a leaky faucet."

"Dr. Harper spoke to me about that call. He was somewhat upset."

"I should say so! That boy was so badly injured, no one would have done him any good. Dr. Kirk tried to take him to the O.R. himself. I set him straight on that, you can be sure."

"Miss Cluny, I certainly appreciate your concern and your outrage—"

"There is something else," she interrupted, before he could dismiss her. "Toward the end, when it should have been obvious that nothing was going to save that unfortunate young man, Dr. Kirk rushed out to his car and came back with a case of intravenous packets of five hundred cubic centimeters each. They contained a creamy fluid. I thought it was a form of plasma."

"You thought? Didn't he tell you?"

"He would answer none of my questions. Just refused to give me information and pressured one of our nurses, Esperanza Gomez, into transfusing the boy with it. It wasn't five minutes after we had pumped the fluid into the boy that he went into cardiac arrest. After he was pronounced dead, I took one of the empty packets.

"The packets had University identification markings on them. I called a friend of mine who works in one of the labs there where they are conducting research in blood disorders and blood chemistry. She told me that Dr. Kirk has been working on an artificial blood. They've used it on dogs and now he has applications in to get permission to test it on humans. But he couldn't wait, you see. He had the material with him and he saw an opportunity for using it on that boy. He saw the boy was dying and decided to do a little experimentation. That's what he did, Mr. Anthony. He used a dying boy as a guinea pig."

Anthony smiled broadly at the old nurse. Lovely, he thought. Just lovely. What a pissing contest this is going to be. He picked up the phone. "Get me payroll," he said when his secretary answered.

Cluny shifted uncomfortably in her chair. If she comes forward one more inch, Anthony thought even as he maintained his smile, she's going to fall right on her ass.

"This is Mr. Anthony," he said when he had his connection. "Can you give me the years of service and salary status for Gloria Cluny?" The shifting in the chair before him continued.

"Ah," he said when he had his answer. "I don't believe that is adequate for someone who has been with us for that long. Add seventy-five dollars a week to that, would you, starting immediately." He hung up and came out from behind the desk. "Miss Cluny," he said, "it's been a pleasure."

He waited until she had closed the door behind her before he picked up the receiver on his private line and punched out the number for Harrison Cummings.

Two hours later a motorboat pulled out of the St. Francis Yacht Club near Fisherman's Wharf and bounced gently away until it was well into open water. Harrison Cummings, the hospital's attorney and Anthony's own legal adviser, took a quick inventory of the other craft in the bay. Because it was a weekday there were only a few "rag" skippers, as Cummings liked to call sailboat owners. Cummings rubbed his hands together then slammed down on the gearshift. The twin engines roared into action and the forty-two-foot white power cruiser, as thin and pointed as an arrowhead, skipped into the air and raced away along the water's surface. Anthony had gone out with Cummings often and now, as before, he was not sure whether he was thrilled or petrified as the boat, skipping, diving, and swerving, streaked to its destination, a small island across the Bay. It was an isolated place and whenever Anthony and Cummings had anything important to talk about, they headed, equipped with fishing gear, jugs full of martinis, a basket replete with sandwiches, to the lee side of the island. Many of Anthony's best maneuvers had been refined and been guaranteed the sanctity of the law there.

They swept around the island and found their favored spot. Cummings cut the engines and cast the anchor. With only a few perfunctory curses for minor obstacles, Cummings and Anthony prepared in dead earnest for the afternoon ahead. Cummings set out the corned-beef sandwiches, the pickles, cole slaw, and, of course, the now very cold Beefeater martinis. Meanwhile, Anthony sorted through the fishing gear and prepared lines and bait for them both. Only when they had done a thorough inventory of their preparations did they settle down to their conversation.

"Did you reread the article?" Anthony asked.

"Yeah," Cummings answered from behind a mouthful of sandwich. "Interesting kid, that Kirk."

"Interesting, my ass. The bastard is dangerous."

"Dangerous?"

"He's after our patients, Harrison. He got himself appointed head of a new trauma department at the University and now he's obviously launching a campaign to get more patients for his service and to do it at the expense of community institutions like Coit Hill."

"Academics talk like that, Al. Forget about it."

"Don't bet on it. Now that Kirk has himself a little trauma department over there, he has to look for more than his share of patients. If you think helicopters are expensive to maintain, you should take a look at the books for a trauma center sometime. What he aims to do is to paint all the community hospitals as places where they operate on trauma patients with rusty kitchen knives and then siphon off all that business for himself."

"So you propose . . ."

"To go after his ass. We've put a lot of money into that chopper of ours. I don't need anyone badmouthing it or campaigning against it. I certainly don't want the board of supervisors or some bureaucrat to get the idea there's reason to shut the operation down."

"Oh, hell, Al, you're just being paranoid. No one can tell you not to fly that thing. Not to fly ten of them if you wanted to. As your attorney I'll guarantee your right to put in a trauma service."

"I'm not so sure that it's just paranoia. I want to put a stop to it now, before it gets out of hand." Anthony stared glumly out at the waters and his slack line, as if the fish below the surface were also part of a conspiracy to thwart him.

Cummings laughed. "Come on, lighten up. You're blowing the whole thing out of proportion. You want my two hundred dollars an hour worth of advice? Leave it be. Who the hell is Kirk? Who ever heard of him before, who will ever hear of him again? If you keep still now, he'll fade into oblivion. If you dignify his little tirade with a response, it will just add fuel to the flames."

"Kirk is not the kind of pest that fades away!" Anthony's fishing pole, propped into its holder on the rail, bent forward now and he leaped to take it in hand. After a brief struggle he reeled in a baby shark. Disgusted, he freed his hook and threw the fish back in the water. "I made some calls after Cluny left the office. Word has it he's a zealot. He works day and night on his trauma teams. He's written multiple papers for journals on trauma care. Whenever studies are published about death rates among trauma patients, in the next issue or two there'll be a letter from A. Kirk, M.D., discussing the implications of the study or the moral behind it. I mean, he's a nut on the subject."

"If he's such a hotshot, what's he doing moonlighting at your place?"

"Who knows? Maybe he needs the dough. He sure as shit isn't getting rich on an assistant professor's salary. More probably, that son of a bitch is trying to gather information on us. The man could be dangerous." Anthony slammed down his fishing rod. "We've got nothing to hide. I'll stack up the care we give patients with any hospital around here."

Cummings, who had just finished his second martini, said nothing for a few minutes, concentrating instead on his corned-beef sandwich. He lifted the top piece of rye bread and looked on the thick layer of meat as if he were gazing at the backside of one of the young boys he was known to favor. The adoration over, he spread mustard and a generous dollop of cole slaw on the meat and replaced the bread. He took a generous bite and chewed it slowly.

"Why don't you give him what he wants?" he said after he had swallowed.

"Are you nuts?"

"Aren't you chairman, or something, of the committee that advises the board of supervisors on things like paramedic training?"

"It's more than that. It's the Joint Committee for Emergency Services. We give them good advice on a number of emergency medicine issues."

"I'm sure the advice they get from you is excellent. Here's what I have in mind. Announce that the committee has considered Kirk's views and that it is concerned about their implications. Call a public meeting of the committee where, you'll say, you'll give Kirk an opportunity to ventilate his concerns. Make it look as if you really want to listen to what he has to say. By the way, you do control the committee, don't you?"

"Yeah."

"Good. Agree beforehand with your cronies what kind of measures you can announce that would make it seem that you are trying to meet some of his concerns but that would not do a great deal of violence to your way of doing business. Then, after his speech, announce them. Presto. You've cut his balls off by taking the initiative away from him. Your committee and the community hospitals will come out smelling like roses because it'll look as if you are all trying to grapple with the issues he has raised."

"Harry . . ."

"It'll work, Al."

"And if it doesn't?"

Cummings put down his sandwich. "Why then, we'll have a whole lot of surprises for our good Dr. Kirk. A whole lot."

7

The greetings as he wandered into the hospital were cool, almost perfunctory: a "Good morning" or even a shortened "Morning," followed by a quick tight smile. Maybe it's my imagination, Allan said to himself at first, maybe that's the way we all act early in the morning every day and today I'm more conscious of it because of the story. Yet, as the morning wore on, it became increasingly clear to him that the coolness was not something his mind had conjured up.

When he asked nurses for patient records, they were put on the counter in front of him without comment. When he sought further information on how a patient had done during the night, the facts were passed on in clipped, dry fashion. The clear chill frightened Allan because he knew that the reception he was receiving was not an indication of the personal feelings the women harbored, but an indication of the way in which the people in power at the hospital felt about him. As seismographs capable of sensing the most minute of tremors in the hospital's political crust, nurses were without parallel. A dozen of them strategically placed along the San Andreas Fault, he had laughingly told himself on those occasions when he had been able to watch their reactions to others who had strayed, would neatly solve California's need for an accurate earthquake prediction system.

Allan soon found confirmation that the nursing staff had read correctly the shock waves set off by the Younger article. Not one physician stopped him in the halls for an impromptu discussion of any medical problem. No one came over to kid with him when he stopped by the physicians' lounge to fill his coffee mug. Physicians with whom he had to discuss the trauma patients still in ICU or who had moved on to conventional rooms were civil and polite. But the feeling of camaraderie, of colleagues battling a common foe, was missing. Every doctor with whom he consulted, it seemed to Allan, answered his every question as if he had stopped a stranger on the street and had asked directions to the nearest public bathroom.

Worst of all, when he walked up to Dorr's office, hoping to talk things out, his secretary curtly told him that Dorr would be in meetings all day but had left a message that Allan was to be in the chief of staff's office at 5:30 that afternoon.

As he slowly walked away from Dorr's office, cries of "Leper! Leper! Clear the road" bounced off his back. Turning around, he saw David Fedder coming up behind him, grinning broadly.

"Thanks, Fedder," Allan greeted him. "Just what I need."

"Hey. Just a little humor to lighten things up. Really getting the deep freeze, huh?"

"It's warmer on Saturn. What do you hear?"

"The rumor mill is going crazy," Fedder said, enjoying the opportunity to pass along the gossip. "The talk is that all the funding for the trauma program is going to be withdrawn. Some say the money will stay but that the program is going to be folded back into surgery. Others think the money will stay, the program will stay independent, but that you're about to be fired. The residents are afraid that if the program is shut down they won't be able to get in anywhere else because of what you're doing. And, of course, every one is saying how they love and admire you, but that this time you've gone too far."

"So how come you're talking to me?"

"Oh, you know, that old Jewish instinct for taking the side of the downtrodden."

Allan laughed, thankful for the younger man's show of support. "Well, enough of this crap," Allan said, trying to sound cheerful. "Let's go see some patients and get some work done. Anything interesting go on last night? No one will tell me anything but the most basic stuff."

"We do have one hassle on the male ward. The old 'Rule of the Cock' is giving us trouble again. Come see."

Nine of the ten beds in the male ward were open to view, their inhabitants either sleeping or watching television. A curtain was drawn around the tenth bed. Fedder, with a nod of his head, bade Allan follow him through an opening in the sheet.

For the briefest of moments Allan was confused. The patient lying on top of the sheets was a tall, startlingly beautiful woman. Her face, though long, was graceful and her large brown eyes, set wide apart, were more round than oval. Her lips were smooth, their outlines drawn precisely, the perfect models for a lipstick ad. Her wavy blonde hair fell neatly about her face.

"Shit!" was her greeting.

"Yes, nice seeing you too, Miss Janetta," Fedder said. "How's it going this morning?"

"How d'you *think* it's going? You got me locked up behind this curtain like I was some kinda freak. Having to ring up the nurse every time I have to pee."

"Is it unreasonable for me to ask what's going on?" Allan broke in.

"Miss Janetta here is not exactly a miss."

"I sure am. I—"

Fedder held up his hand. "Miss Janetta, as she prefers to be known, came into the E.R. last night about, what, seven?"

The woman nodded, folded her arms, and looked away, disgusted at the thought of having to listen to the whole story again.

"She had a pretty good gash on the inside of her left thigh. Seems that a customer who was not quite as drunk as she thought he was took offense when he found that for his fifty bucks he was getting a handful of cock instead of what he was expecting. They got into a fight, the john whipped out a knife, and offered to help her meet truth-in-advertising laws. Lucky for her, she got her leg up in time."

"Shit. I've been taking my hormones, got rid of my beard, got these." She cupped one well-shaped breast in each hand. "I sure am a woman."

"Not with that nine-inch dong hanging there you're not."

"It ain't no nine inches." She was honestly offended. "Six more tricks, and I'll have all the money for that operation too."

"In any case," Fedder went on, addressing Allan. "We stitched her up and sent her up here. But some of the guys here suddenly are not quite as sick as they seem. Two of them tried to get into bed with her. One guy followed her into the can."

"Did I complain?"

Allan ignored her. "Did you consider sending her to the female ward?"

"Of course I considered it. The supervising nurse had a hemorrhage when I told her."

"Private beds?"

"There's a severe burn case in one, a guy with DTs so bad he was upsetting the whole ward in the second, and that bank VP that came in after the car accident two weeks ago."

"Isn't he ready for transfer to his private hospital?"

"No. He's still too unstable."

Allan pulled up the transsexual's nightgown and gingerly began to pick out the gauze packing that had been inserted into the deep thigh wound. Bloody fluid oozed out. "He's going to need vigorous care for that," Allan said. "Some antibiotics for a couple of days and maybe some whirlpool treatments should do it." Allan put his hand on the patient's shoulder. "You're just going to have to piss in your pot in here until you're ready for discharge. But tell you what. Maybe we can get you a TV in here. That should tide you over."

The interlude with the transsexual proved to be the only relief from the tedium that came with his ostracism. He ate lunch alone. Though he doggedly insisted on going to the small coffee-and-cake farewell for a German physician who had been in the surgery department as a fellow for a year, he left after ten minutes when it became obvious that his presence was casting a pall over the affair. When 5:30 finally arrived and he went off to see Dorr, he felt as if he had been in solitary confinement in San Quentin for a month.

As Allan sat before him, Dorr made an almost exaggerated show of reading the Younger story. "Quite a little speech," he said. "Well?"

"What can I say, Phil? I got caught. The stuff about Coit Hill was a two-minute conversation in a twenty-minute interview. He caught me off guard."

"It wouldn't be quite so easy to catch you off guard if you learned to think a little bit." Dorr folded the paper and threw it back on the desk. "My phone started ringing at 6:15 this morning, Allan. And not one of those calls, I'm sure you won't be surprised to find out, was from anyone who thought you deserved a medal. People are exceedingly upset. Exceedingly upset."

Allan flared, the day's frustration welling up in him.

"What the hell is everyone so pissed about? I didn't say that *we* were doing a shitty job. I didn't run down this institution."

"No, that you didn't do. But that's not the point. In the first place you ran down fellow doctors. Most people around here have always thought you were off the wall, but they were willing to put up with you because they consider you a pretty goddamn good physician. But this is different, Allan. This tells them not just that you are of a different mold but that you are a renegade. This warns them that the next time they see you quoted in the press, it may be because you may have something to say about them."

"That's ridiculous."

"Is it? What happens the next time a cardiologist doesn't respond as quickly as you want with a consult on a trauma patient who has a severe complercardiac arrhythmia? You going to tell Younger about it? I'm not saying you will, just that that is what they think.

"And that's not the worst of it. You're young but you didn't fall off a cabbage truck yesterday. A lot of your colleagues work here because they love this kind of work. But they depend on the docs on the outside to refer patients to them. It's the cases that are referred here from the community hospitals that are the tough and challenging ones, the kind that make University work interesting, exciting, and give us the opportunity to come up with better treatments. When you disparage community doctors, the people here see those referrals dry up."

"Oh, hell, Phil, where are they going to send them?"

"UC-Davis, Stanford. Even UCLA. You'd be surprised how far people will travel if they think a University genius will do them some good. In any case, the doctors here are the least of it. Your friend, the administrator, is beside himself. Do you have any idea how many indigent patients community hospitals refer to us in addition to the tough cancers, the metabolic cases, or the autoimmune puzzles?"

"The transfers? The dumps?"

"They may be dumps to you but to this hospital they are money. This hospital bills the county and the state for a hell of a lot of money for care to indigents. The private hospitals scorn those patients because the government pays far less than one hundred percent for their care, but that money is an important part of this institution's bank account. And now you've gone and put the hex on that too."

"You mean that bean counter upstairs is afraid that Coit Hill isn't going to send us any more of their discards? Are they going to send them to Stanford too?"

"No, they won't send the indigents to Stanford. But Anthony will find a way of hurting us with them, you watch and see. Or at least that's what the 'bean counter' thinks. And now, my friend, for the real surprise."

Allan steeled himself, sure he was going to hear that the hospital board had changed its mind and was withdrawing his appointment to head the trauma department.

"Anthony called me about an hour ago."

"What did he ask for, my head?"

"That's what I was fully prepared for. But no, he was as smooth and unctuous as he could be. He said he was quite concerned about your feelings about Coit Hill and the other community hospitals. He was wondering, he said, if he could approach you about appearing before the Joint Committee for Emergency Services he heads so that some of these things could be, as he put it, 'aired in the appropriate forum.'"

"Then why all that lecturing about how what I said to Younger is going to endanger everyone's livelihood around here? Obviously it didn't bother him half as much as it bothered my friends around here."

"Allan. Allan. Allan. In the first place, what would you expect me to do? Put out a general memo saying 'Anthony forgives Kirk'? In the second place, I smell something suspicious. I think Anthony is setting you up for something, though I'm not exactly sure what."

"So you don't think I should go."

"Quite the contrary. You have to go. You see, that's part of the trap. If you turn down the invitation, all he has to do is point out at the meeting, loudly and clearly, that you were given a chance to present your views, but that you declined and that all you were obviously interested in was publicity for yourself and the University."

"And if I go?"

"Then you'll be center stage. Just like the lady tied, spread-eagle, to a spinning board while her partner throws long, sharp knives ten minutes after they've had a fight. If I were you I would be very well prepared for that meeting."

"I'll be prepared all right. I haven't mentioned it before but for the last few weeks I've been putting in time at the medical examiner's office, looking for autopsies and records on people who died in community hospitals after trauma."

"With an eye toward doing what?"

"Analyzing the cases and seeing how many people might have been saved if they had had adequate trauma care. I haven't got quite enough cases yet, nor have I done the statistical work, but I don't see any reason why I shouldn't have it done for presentation at the meeting."

"You wouldn't dare!"

"Why not, Phil? If I have hard facts they can't be interpreted as just another temper tantrum. Maybe if those people actually see evidence about the care people are receiving in those emergency rooms, they'll stop fighting the notion that we need a full-fledged trauma system."

"Those people don't want facts. They just want to be left alone to enjoy the status quo. They're not out looking for anything that will complicate their lives. Moreover, no study you do and present in that fashion will convince anyone of anything. Just the fact that you are doing it will be enough to discredit it in their eyes."

"So you think I'm wasting my time?"

"Not necessarily. Do the study, do all the statistical work, and then submit it to a journal that has an editorial board that critiques submissions. If they accept it and publish it, then it will be much more effective as a tool toward whatever it is you want to do. In case I haven't made myself clear: under no circumstances bring it up at the meeting. In fact, I'll go even further. Under no circumstances make it public until it has been published in an acceptable journal."

Dorr rose. "Arrange for Santorre to cover your schedule for a few days. Clear your head, prepare yourself, at least psychologically, for your meeting with Anthony." Dorr stopped. Allan saw that he was trying to find a way to take some of the edge off the scolding he had delivered. "Son, you're a valuable member of this University. Be careful at the meeting. Now get out of here, I've got patients to see."

Allan drove around aimlessly, not wanting really to go anywhere, not wanting to go home. He drove up the winding narrow streets leading to Twin Peaks. He felt a momentary pang of jealousy when his eyes fell on the low wall where Julie and Jim had made love. A vision of the lovers began to form in his mind, but he suppressed the thought, concentrating instead on the vista before him. A pink hue suffused the city. The pastel lighting softened the outline of the city's hills and even managed to give warmth to the scores of towering office buildings that had been thrown up in the financial district. The noise of the city didn't reach him up here and he felt as if he were looking at his own, private diorama.

Glad he had driven up, but still filled with turmoil, he stepped back into his car. An hour later, not quite sure of the route he had taken, he was parking on Sutro Heights, the palisades high above the Pacific Ocean on the city's west side. He walked slowly past

Cliff House, which contained a seafood restaurant, boutiques, and gift shops, and looked down at the ocean, now at low tide, and the jumble of small rocks and large boulders. He zipped up the jacket he had put on and wound his way down the trail leading from Sutro Heights to the shore below. Stepping carefully on small boulders exposed by the receding tide, he made his way out to the largest rock accessible to him and sat down. This was his place, the one spot where, sensing the pull and power of the ocean, he could in absolute privacy think out his most profound questions.

But now he was feeling little in the way of relief. Though he still had a good deal of work to do on his study, what he had found so far, combined with his personal experiences and the stories told him by fellow residents who had worked at other community hospitals, convinced him that unnecessary deaths were occurring in emergency rooms every day. It was a problem so significant he could not, as an individual, ignore it. As he thought of Dorr's instruction to keep quiet about his findings and beliefs, he grew angrier and angrier; he determined not to follow the chief of staff's advice. But that thought, too, depressed him. If he continued with his research at the medical examiner's office in order to find enough cases to convince even the greatest skeptic and if he went public with his charges, Allan knew, he would be on a direct collision course with Dorr, who had been a valued mentor throughout the last six years, and a man he admired and loved. He lingered on the rock, finally deciding that he would say nothing about his study when he faced the Joint Committee, but that he would do something to bring it into the public eye if he saw that the medical community refused to deal with the trauma problem. Having set his course, he rose and, somewhat saddened by his decision to cast himself away from Dorr, made his way back to the parking lot and drove home.

Without bothering to turn on the living-room light, he went directly into the kitchen and opened the refrigerator, its bulb casting a pale, yellowish light over the otherwise dark room, and rummaged through the shelves, looking for something to eat. Nothing appealed to him. He walked back to the living room and switched on the light. The room, with its high ceiling, the broad bay window with its bits and pieces of stained glass and leadwork, and the shiny pegged and grooved hardwood floor, always warmed him, made him feel glad to be home. Now it seemed perversely desolate. He walked around, picked up a newspaper here, a book there. In desperation he scanned the TV guide's late movie listings.

He turned off the ceiling light and made his way to his desk in the corner of the room, and switched on the large lamp clamped to the desk's side. Its powerful beam instantly spread across the paper-cluttered desktop. When writing for a journal or researching a difficult case, he liked to work like this. The spotlight on the desk reminded him of the operating room, of the strong white light that focused his attention on the patient supine before him.

He shuffled through the papers, the journals that had come in during the last ten days, the copies of articles he had torn out of older magazines. He leafed through three journals, found nothing of interest in them, and threw them in the general direction of the wastebasket. Two hit their target. The third landed with a heavy thump on the floor. He looked through the articles, sorted them into piles according to subject matter, then scanned the papers, threw some away, put others into a neat pile.

Satisfied now with the pristine appearance of the desk, he turned back to his filing cabinet and found the four folders containing the data he had been gathering in the medical examiner's office. Since the night that Julie had dragged him off to the county fair, he had been able to get back to the M.E.'s file room three times and had found another dozen cases in which trauma patients had died in community-hospital operating and emergency rooms or in ICUs. After looking quickly through the folders, he grabbed his jacket, snapped off the light, and bolted out the door. Twenty minutes later, under the sterile glare of the fluorescent lighting, he was hard at work in the medical examiner's file room.

He was perched high on the rolling ladder when he heard the footsteps approaching, stopping at the door. There was a second or two of silence before the door slowly opened. He watched as Julie walked to the worktable. She picked up a file, looked through it, put it down, picked up another one. Puzzled by the silence, she looked around.

"Allan?"

He considered saying nothing, of making it seem that though he had been there, he had already left. "Over here."

She looked to her right and up. "Hi."

"Hi."

"Making any progress?"

"Some."

"Will you come down and be civil or am I going to have to get a sore neck standing here talking up to you?"

He came down and walked back to the table, Julie following. "I'm just not sure that there is anything to talk about."

"This," she replied as she pointed at the folders. "Us."

"This I can finish myself. Us? I should have taken you at your word when you said there couldn't be anything between us. As for what happened, I'm sorry I overstepped my bounds."

"You couldn't have overstepped your bounds if I hadn't erased them a bit myself. I know what I said when we first met, Allan. It was a knee-jerk reaction."

"And that scene on the couch. How would you classify that reaction?"

"Don't be such a bastard, Allan! I'm trying to tell you something. I've grown to like you. A lot. Enough to have wanted to make love with you. I thought I could. . . . I thought if I could finally get over Jim, it would be with you."

"So you tried your little experiment and found out you couldn't."

"Goddamn you!" Her eyes were moistening. "Why do you insist on believing that you are the only one with feelings? I was as surprised by my reaction as you were. It scared me. It frightened the hell out of me."

She took his hand. He successfully fought the impulse to withdraw it. For the first time since she had come in, he looked directly into her face. Her lips were slightly parted. Her cheeks were flushed. There was a plea in her eyes and he did not resist. He reached out and gathered her into his arms.

"Julie," he finally said, pushing her back so he could look at her. "Don't take this wrong. I see this sort of thing all the time.

Two people get in an accident and one dies. The other one goes through hell feeling guilty about having survived. You won't get over Jim until you get over those feelings. It's not your fault that you are alive and that he is dead."

"I know it's not my fault I survived." The tears were spilling out now. "But it is my fault he died. He had a little sports car I loved to drive. *I* was behind the wheel. *I* lost control of the car. *I* killed him."

Allan drew her toward him and held her tightly. "No, you didn't do that either, Julie. You were driving and were in an accident in which he died. But that doesn't make it your fault. You could just as well be angry with him for not wearing a seat belt or for not warning you about whatever idiosyncrasy in that car made it hard to handle on a winding, downhill street." She burrowed into him, seeking refuge from herself. Then she pulled back and clasped her hands behind his neck. "Make love to me, Allan. Please."

He didn't move.

"Please." She leaned forward and kissed him, picked up the files he had scattered on the table and put them on one of the chairs. Kissing gently, unwilling to pull apart, they made their way onto the tabletop. They caressed each other slowly, kissed and nuzzled. They freed each other of shirts, jeans, undergarments and, without yet consummating their desire, pressed against each other. Carefully, Allan ran his fingertips down her spine and over her buttocks. He cupped his hand and, reaching, caressed the inside of her thigh. As she responded, he brought his hand to the top of her leg, then slowly upward.

"Allan," she whispered in his ear, "no more screaming. You don't have to be so careful. Promise."

She opened her legs and he moved onto her, slipping easily into her, and she pushed up to meet him. They moved back and forth to a slow-motion beat, straining only to keep their bodies as close together as possible. Their release came slowly, a long gentle wave.

Allan kissed her eyelids, her nose, her lips, then drew back to study her. Julie smiled, then opened her eyes. She regarded him for a moment, then laughed. "If you are expecting me to say thank you, forget it."

He traced the outline of her face with his index finger, then bent his head and kissed her. "A sigh of contentment would be enough."

Julie reached up to tweak his nose, but he twisted away. He looked at the clock on the wall. "It's close to three o'clock," he said. "Let's go find somewhere to have breakfast, then go home and get some sleep. What do you say?"

"Not hungry yet. Why don't we look for some more cases, then go eat?" She paused. "Anyway, what do you mean, get breakfast go home to sleep? Don't you have to go back to the hospital?"

"I'm not going back to the hospital."

Alarmed, she sat up. "What happened? Did they fire you?"

He laughed, then filled her in on the previous day's events.

"And you are going to accept Anthony's invitation?"

"I don't see that I have much choice. I'm damned if I do and I'm damned if I don't." With a groan he rolled off the table, found his pants, and put them on. "Gads, that's hard on the old knees."

"I don't know what you're complaining about. At least you were on top." She rose as well, flexing and rolling her shoulders. "Are you going to say anything about the study?"

"I'm under orders not to. I told Dorr about it and he told me in no uncertain terms that I'd be a fool to bring it up at the meeting. I'll give him that, Julie, but not much more."

In the days that followed, Julie and Allan sometimes worked individually in the file room, but more often they worked together. As they made their way through rack after rack of records, the number of deaths Allan wanted to include in his study grew. When they had amassed one hundred cases, they went to a supermarket, bought food, and then locked themselves into Julie's apartment. Julie began to prepare formulations for the statistics they would need. Allan, meanwhile, studied and analyzed each case, carefully reading all the notes and reports supplied to the medical examiner's office by the hospital. He scrutinized each autopsy report, down to the smallest detail.

"What do you think?" Julie asked late one night as they were savoring a bottle of wine as a reward for the day's diligence.

"Not much yet. I've gone through only sixty-three cases so far. Ask me tomorrow night. I'll be done then." He unbuttoned the top of the men's pajamas she was wearing and helped her out of her panties. He then reached for the bottle of wine and, starting at Julie's throat, began emptying its contents on her body, taking care to save a generous portion for her pubic hair, her thighs, and the flesh between them.

Julie giggled as Allan began licking the liquid from the small indentation in her throat. The laughter, though, subsided quickly as he lapped at her breasts, her abdomen. Her breath quickened as he drew on one thigh, brushed his mouth lightly over her mound of Venus on the way to the other thigh. Even as he lingered there she began to undulate rhythmically.

As Allan moved his mouth back to her center, he heard a husky "turn around." He did and as he brought his thighs to her face, he could first feel her breath, then her taking him in. Placing his hands on her buttocks, he pulled her toward him, kissing her, flicking his tongue with increasing ardor as her attentions to him grew more insistent. Allan felt himself hurtling to his finish and tried to pull away from her mouth. But Julie held him tightly, simultaneously pushing herself against his face. They rocked harder and harder. A powerful shudder passed through her, then a second and a third. Her rapid-sequence convulsions excited him beyond endurance. When her fourth orgasm burst over her, he relinquished control.

Exhausted by the intensity of their work and their interludes of sex, they sat side by side in front of Julie's home computer. Julie was leaning back on her chair, her arms crossed over her breasts, wearing her satisfaction like a velvet glove. Allan was bent forward, elbows on his knees, chin resting on his fists.

"And there, Dr. Kirk, you have it. Forty-seven of the one hundred patients who died in community emergency rooms after having been involved in some sort of an accident could have been saved. Thirty-six of the forty-seven died because they did not get the surgical intervention they needed. The average delay in getting these people to an operating room was two-point-five hours. Twenty percent of those who died unnecessarily died because the nature of their wounds was misdiagnosed.

"Now here's some really neat stuff," Julie added, punching a key and calling some new statistics to the screen. "Fifty-eight percent of the patients who died because they were not taken to surgery at all, or only after long delays, died between eleven P.M. and four A.M. Thirty percent died on a Saturday or a Sunday. Only twelve percent died during regular business hours when hospitals could presumably get their hands on surgeons. And, finally, look at this. Sixty percent of the deaths occurred in what we consider large hospitals, the big institutions everyone holds in awe."

Allan got up and stretched. "We're going to have to use that material, Julie. We're going to have to use it."

The scene that greeted him as he walked into the meeting room where the Joint Committee for Emergency Services had scheduled its gathering did nothing to allay the qualms Allan had felt about conforming with Anthony's request. Seated behind a long table set up on the dais were some of San Francisco's most powerful medical people. At the table's far right sat the physician who headed one of San Francisco's emergency room physicians groups. His doctors were under contract to a dozen hospitals in the Bay area. He was brilliant and well versed in even the smallest of nuances in emergency medicine and the delivery of emergency care. But he also fought hard to maintain the status quo, one that allowed his group to earn millions of dollars a year. A sound percentage of those earnings, moreover, found their way into the campaign treasuries of three of the county's supervisors. No proposed change in San Francisco's emergency-care network ever affected him adversely.

Next to the emergency-room entrepreneur sat the county fire chief, the man who had been given authority to supervise the city's paramedic organization; then came the representative from the

Northern California Hospital Council, a man who until a few months earlier had been a bureaucrat in the county's Health and Welfare Services Department and whose job at the department had been to monitor emergency services provided by the city's private hospitals. Next to him sat Anthony, fiddling with his gavel, looking, as usual, as if he had just stepped out of the pages of *Gentlemen's Quarterly*. Hard at Anthony's elbow was a neurosurgeon whose image of himself was immense, even for someone in his specialized field. (Prior to assuming the chairmanship of the neurosurgery department at one of the city's largest hospitals, the specialist had been an adjunct professor of neurosurgery at the University. The appointment was canceled after one year because he had refused even the most senior of residents the right to operate on the brain. "Only I touch the brain!" he would shout at the residents who assisted him. "Only *I* touch the brain.")

"Jesus," Allan whispered to Julie, who had decided at the last minute to come with him, "talk about an invitation to a hanging."

"Just keep cool, Allan." She clasped his right hand in both of hers as they sat down.

At precisely 7 P.M., Anthony pounded his gavel on the table and called the meeting to order.

"Dr. Kirk?" Anthony looked around, not quite sure which of the few people in the audience he should be addressing. Allan stood up.

Anthony flashed a broad, brittle smile. "Thank you so much for coming, doctor. Your presence here is appreciated. For your information, we are going to dispense with the routine matters on the agenda and take up what is really on everyone's mind here, your very interesting thoughts on the state of emergency care in this county." Anthony smiled again. The others just stared at Allan as if they were trying to determine precisely what kind of foul-smelling swamp creature had wandered into their midst.

"To refresh everyone's memory, let me review your public comments." In a clear, crisp voice, speaking slowly and articulating precisely, Anthony read the Younger article from beginning to end. With a flourish he put down the paper.

Hearing Dorr's words echoing in his head, Allan fought to be humble. "Let me assure you, Mr. Anthony, that the article distressed me as much as it did you. My remarks were taken out of context and—"

"Dr. Kirk, somehow everyone's remarks, especially the ones they regret when they see them in black and white, are always taken out of context." It was the emergency entrepreneur talking. "But the fact is, you've scared the hell out of a lot of San Franciscans. People with a cut finger are afraid to go to an E.R. You have impugned the capabilities of a lot of hard-working people."

"I realize that, doctor." Allan almost gagged on his servility. "But what I was trying to say—"

"What you said was that hospitals are knowingly allowing people to bleed to death in the emergency room," interrupted the man from the hospital council.

"Gentlemen," Anthony broke in, looking first to his left, then to his right. "Dr. Kirk is not on trial here. He has some concerns about the delivery of emergency care. We invited him here to air them."

He turned to Allan and again graced him with a generous smile. "Dr. Kirk, we're sure you wouldn't make charges as you did just off the top of your head. Let's begin this way. Do you have any data indicating that there are needless trauma deaths?"

"No, I don't have *direct* evidence. But there have been scattered reports of needless deaths—"

The neurosurgeon cut in. "I've been practicing in this community for twenty years. I've taken E.R. calls for all that time and not once have I seen a death I could call preventable. Never!"

Allan could feel Julie's eyes boring into his back, urging him to retain control.

"There have been scientific studies done elsewhere in the nation showing a high incidence of preventable trauma deaths. San Francisco is no different," Allan said.

"Of course it is different, Dr. Kirk," the fire chief said, talking in the avuncular tone he used on television to explain why he could not hire more women as firefighters or why he sympathized with his men when they demanded special equipment for fighting fires in buildings where AIDS cases had been documented. "San Francisco is different because it is a small city. No trauma patient is ever more than ten minutes from the closest hospital."

"Transport time is not the issue," Allan said, deliberately keeping his voice low.

"Then what is, Dr. Kirk?"

"The issue is what happens once the patient gets to the hospital. That's where the system is breaking down."

The hospital council representative leaned forward. "Let's assume for the moment that you are right, doctor. Just how would you propose to change things?"

"My feeling is that one hospital in this city should be designated a trauma center. It would commit itself to having in-house, twenty-four hours a day, a general surgeon, anesthesiologists, neurosurgeons, O.R. crews, blood-bank facilities. All severely injured patients should be taken to that hospital."

"And of course that hospital would be the one where you practice medicine," the neurosurgeon said. "My, how convenient."

Allan started to respond in kind, but stopped himself. "I'm sure that what we all want in this community is the best care for our patients," he said slowly. "We want the kind of system in which, if one of us or a member of our family were seriously injured, they would have the best chance for survival. Whether it is the University hospital or not is essentially irrelevant."

The neurosurgeon was shaking his head, impatiently waiting for Allan to finish. "Let me ask you this. Someone is run down right in front of my hospital. Now, rather than bring him right into my institution, you would have the Chief's paramedics run him halfway across town to the trauma center—presuming my hospital does not get the designation?"

Allan nodded.

"Well, then, doctor, would you care to guess how many people would die unnecessarily while they were being transported? I mean, how can you possibly justify not taking patients directly to the E.R. of a fine hospital like mine and instead spending twenty minutes fighting traffic to get to your trauma center?"

"Because, as I said before, transport time is not the key. Data in study after study has shown that the few extra minutes spent in transporting patients is well rewarded by taking the patient to a hospital that can resuscitate him in the E.R. and then have him in the operating room for definitive control of bleeding within ten or twelve minutes of his arrival at the hospital."

"Somehow I can't shake the feeling that this is all rather self-serving," the emergency-room entrepreneur chimed in. "We know the University is having major financial problems. Now they've gone out on a limb to develop this trauma program that you are apparently going to head and now they have to figure out a way to pay for it. What it looks like to me is that you are going out into the community to stir up trouble and to divert patients to your E.R."

"I'm sorry then, but I don't understand why you invited me," Allan said. "It seems that you've made up your minds already."

"Come on, doctor, don't be quite so sensitive," Anthony said. "It's true that no one here is keen on a trauma-center system, but that does not mean that we don't want to take your feelings into consideration."

"Which means what?"

"That this committee will recommend to all hospitals that they upgrade their emergency-room procedures. We will recommend that surgeons who fail to respond to two successive calls from the E.R. be dropped from the call list. We'll outline circumstances under which patients with very complex injuries will be transferred to the University after they have been stabilized at the local hospital. Moreover, just today the board of directors at Coit Hill voted to allow other hospitals to use Coit Hill's helicopter for the transportation of difficult trauma patients from their institutions to Coit Hill, if the need arises."

Anthony reached for the pitcher on the table, poured water into his glass, and took a sip. "I have also been authorized, Dr. Kirk, to ask whether you would consider becoming a member of this committee in order to help us carry out these reforms."

Allan felt nausea sweep over him. His voice was low now, not because he wanted to be polite, but because he sensed he had lost the battle. "I am sure the committee will make all of these recommendations," he said. "But since it has no enforcement powers, it seems to me there would be no way of ascertaining whether or not any of the hospitals put your suggestions into play." He stopped for a moment, trying to choose his words. "The suggestion that patients be stabilized in a community hospital and then be sent to the University if the case were to prove 'complex' I find particularly offensive. What that will mean is that the current wallet-biopsy system would be perpetuated. Patients without insurance will be dumped on us. Patients with insurance will not fare much better. They will be run through a vast series of expensive diagnostic tests and procedures and then, if the problems are overwhelming, those patients also would be dumped. And what would be happening meanwhile is that a major portion of the time we have to save the patient would be wasted. The whole thing is a sham, a scheme designed to make it seem that the committee is taking my complaints seriously and has tried to act on them in good conscience."

"Dr. Kirk?" Anthony asked. "Is there really no satisfying you?"

"Mr. Anthony, seeing that the committee has apparently decided to take this route, there doesn't seem much more left for me to say. However, if you are determined to go this course, then I would like to suggest one last thing. The committee should appoint a group of individuals who are not directly involved with the University or the community hospitals and have them serve as an evaluation team to see if your ideas are working."

"Come now, Dr. Kirk," the neurosurgeon shot back. "You are talking about setting up another cumbersome committee, and one probably made up of outsiders to boot, since you talk about people not affiliated with the University or other hospitals, that is going to take up the time of physicians who are already overcommitted. We have proposed a reasonable program and you have no cause to doubt the sincerity of those who would carry it out. We hardly need the kind of supervisory group you seem to be suggesting, that will make sure we are all good little boys and girls."

"I'm sorry, then I could not possibly consider serving on the committee."

"We suggested that as a courtesy to you, Dr. Kirk, not that you deserve it," the emergency-room entrepreneur injected. "We never thought that if you chose to accept the appointment we would be sanctified by your presence."

"We may as well be straightforward here, Kirk," added the neurosurgeon. "You are treading on dangerous ground. You have your whole career ahead of you, fellow, don't compromise it now."

"What is that supposed to mean?" Allan ignored Julie's sharp tug at his hand.

"When you face this committee, you see before you more than one hundred and twenty-five years of experience with emergency medicine. The board of supervisors gave us a mandate to see to it that the needs of the people of this county are well met. And that means that we will not allow anyone to undermine the confidence the people of San Francisco have in the fine hospitals available to them or in the very fine men and women who work there."

"So what you are telling me is that I had better shut up, is that it?" Julie tugged again, a bit harder.

"You can put it in any terms you want. All we are saying is that we will not allow anyone to undermine the mandate with which we are charged."

"You said to be straightforward, so by all means let's be. I am not out to sabotage you, or the other doctors in this community or the hospitals. You all do fine work, great work, marvelous work removing gallbladders, doing coronary bypasses, hysterectomies. But trauma is a different kind of medicine and even many emergency-room docs don't appreciate what's involved in bringing back a patient who should, by all rights, be dead. And if you insist on pretending that there is nothing wrong here, that someone who has been in a crunch on the freeway requires help that is no different from the help given someone who has run a lawnmower over his own foot, then indeed you will be carrying out a mandate.

"What you'll be doing is protecting the financial interests of all your buddies and in the process carrying out a mandate for carnage."

Allan turned on his heels and strode out of the room, Julie behind him, hurrying to catch up.

The third person out of the room was Sam Younger, on his way to the nearest public phone.

"This is Younger," he said when the night assistant city editor answered. "Got a goody for you." He waited while the editor dug up someone to take his story, then began to dictate:

> The county's Joint Committee for Emergency Medical Services would rather protect the financial interests of the medical community than institute a meaningful system to handle badly injured accident victims, Dr. Allan Kirk, head of the University of San Francisco's trauma department, charged last night. . . .

8

Still dressed in a short terry-cloth robe, Harrison Cummings stood in the middle of the living room, reading through the Younger account of the Joint Committee's confrontation with Allan. Anthony, who had phoned forty-five minutes earlier and whom Cummings had invited to breakfast, sat in a leather easy chair, studying his surroundings. He had not been here before, though Cummings had often raved to him about the house, one of the finest examples around, he liked to boast, of "neo-Spanish colonial revivalism."

The arched floor-to-ceiling window afforded Anthony a magnificent and unimpeded view of the ocean. Turning, he swiveled the chair to face the inside of the spacious room. A six-foot fireplace framed by a massive oak mantel dominated one wall. A full cathedral ceiling towered over the room, its vault also fashioned out of old oak. Massive timbers jutted down from various points in the vault and joined, at right angles, beams crossing the lowermost boundary of the ceiling. There were wrought angle irons at every joint where beam met beam. The living room's most prominent pieces of furniture were a large rosewood table inlaid with Danish tiles, a creamy-white sectional sofa, two easy chairs, and the grand piano Cummings's mother had always hoped her son would master. To Anthony's left, a broad arch gave way to the dining room, whose walls were lined with embossed leather and which featured a dining set for twelve. To Anthony's right, a smaller archway led to a hallway and a spiral staircase to the second floor.

Fuckin' fags have all the money, Anthony thought.

Cummings's houseboy came in and announced breakfast. They sat down to eggs Benedict, bacon, sausages, hot sourdough rolls, freshly squeezed orange juice, an assortment of jams and jellies, and a pot of steaming coffee.

"What now, counselor?" Anthony asked from behind a mouthful of eggs.

"Any number of things, Al. The question is, what are your goals? Just what is it you and your Joint Committee want to achieve?"

"Never mind the committee. I'll tell you what I want. I want Kirk and the University out of my hair. I'll tell you something, Harry—"

"I do wish you'd stop with the Harry business."

"Sorry, Harrison. I'll tell you something. Kirk, whether he meant to or not, has set something in motion. And I'll tell you how it will go if we just sit here like a bunch of assholes and do nothing. Younger is going to do more stories because that whore just loves sexy stories like trauma centers. Then the *Mirror* will pick it up and shove it to the *Telegraph*, by exhuming bodies of trauma victims or something weird like that, and run headlines that say, 'From the Grave: Questions about Medical Care in San Francisco.' Then those dimwits at the TV stations will decide that they have to get in on the act because nothing draws audiences better than a lot of real-life blood and gore and ambulances running around, lights flashing, sirens screaming.

"And I'll bet you a month's supply of grade-A coke that in no time at all, Kirk, his ivory-tower buddies, half the regents, and a state assemblyman or senator will be leaning mighty heavily on those intellectual dwarfs at the county Board of Supervisors to give the University the trauma-center designation. That is what I think will happen."

Cummings, whose eyes had lit up at the mention of the word "coke," was leaning back in his chair, enjoying the tirade immensely.

"This is not funny, Harrison!" Anthony yelled.

"You're right, you're right. Sorry. What makes you think that the supervisors won't buy the plan you tried to sell last night about upgrading emergency services in every hospital?"

"Because under the steamroller that could get going, upgrading services won't be fancy enough. Kirk already started whining that no one could be sure that under our proposal hospitals were really going to do what they had promised to do. And basically he's right. There would be meetings, everyone would solemnly swear to take better care of crunch victims, they'd do it for about a month, and then it would be back to business as usual. No, with Kirk and Younger raising a lot of hell what we are going to get is a full-blown, bona fide trauma center. The question is just going to be which facility gets the designation."

"And you want to make sure that it's not the University that gets the designation."

"I want that designation, Harrison."

"And to do that you want to get rid of Kirk."

"Precisely. But first we go after the University. They are on shaky financial ground over there. If we can hurt them financially, they won't have the dough to let Kirk's trauma department get bigger than it is now. Once that goes by the wayside, it won't be much harder to get rid of Kirk altogether. There's no other hospital that could give us a run for the designation. Not if they are honest in assessing what they have and what we have."

Cummings took a sip of coffee and spread a heavy layer of strawberry jam on half a sourdough roll. "One way to do that, I suppose, would be for you to have a little chat with other hospital administrators and suggest you all stop referring people to the University. Determine that until the University agrees not to vie for the trauma-center designation, you don't send over the patients they need and want for their work over there. Of course, there is no need to mention to your fellow administrators that the ultimate beneficiary of the pressure on the University will be Coit

Hill. There's no use burdening them with information they don't need."

"Fine idea, except for one thing. The patients the University wants and needs, like the rare cancers or the five-hundred-gram premature babies, are the very patients we don't want to deal with, patients we have to send over whether we like it or not. I can't see Providence or Saint Helena's or anyone suddenly keeping those patients just to put a little heat on the University. No one is going to risk a malpractice suit for the sake of tearing a piece out of Kirk's hide."

They stopped talking when the houseboy came in to clear the table.

"Well, they can always refer those cases to other university hospitals around here," Cummings said after the young man had retreated. "But let's think about something else. The University has a three-million-dollar contract with the county to provide care to indigents not covered by Medi-Cal or Medicare, right?"

"Yeah."

"Any idea when the contract is up?"

"September, I think. I heard someone say that they were already starting to negotiate the next one, that the University wants a ten-percent increase but that the county wants to reduce the contract."

"There you are. Write up a proposal and offer to assume the county contract for ten percent less, for two-point-seven million dollars or, heck, for even less, two-point-five million."

Anthony's face lit up. "You know, Harry—Harrison— sometimes you really earn your money. Son of a bitch! Ninety percent of those people just come in for routine stuff anyway, like runny noses, minor bone fractures, that sort of shit. We could even make money on the deal. I've got a folio full of applications from Pakistani, Indian, and Vietnamese doctors just dying to start their practices here. We can hire them for half the price the University has to pay its docs and have them just take care of the indigent population. I bet we could even put a good public-relations sheen on it. Damn, that's good."

Cummings, ignoring Anthony's enthusiasm, stared off into

space for a while. "You know," he said finally. "Maybe we shouldn't hit them one at a time, first the University, then Kirk. Maybe we should use both barrels of the shotgun at the same time."

"Why?"

"Well, because it seems to me that just taking the University on first might achieve the opposite effect. They might just dig their heels in and fight back. After all, rumor has it, and I think it's fairly accurate, that they have lost half of their cardiac work to the unit you started after you hired Harper away from them. If they see themselves losing yet another service to you, they might just call in a few chits. Like it or not, the University has produced a hell of a lot of doctors in the state, many of whom are very active politically and who could be recruited to help if the University felt it was in real danger."

"So what would you do?"

"Hit them as we talked about, but hit at Kirk at the same time. Make him a very definite liability. Make it difficult and costly for the University to defend itself and Kirk at the same time. Force them first to divvy up their resources for a two-front war, then push it home to them that the only way they could possibly hold their own would be to rid themselves of Kirk. They won't do it right away, but eventually they will. Once they've scuttled him, they will, in effect, have gutted their trauma service. You can then go after the trauma designation and forget the idea of the county contract and let the University go on with that. Everybody will be happy."

"Let me think on that. But if we do go ahead against Kirk at the same time, where do we start? The lawsuit?"

"Precisely. I took all your records on that boy who got the artificial blood to two surgeons I use as consultants. They looked at a copy of the autopsy report. They interviewed Cluny and did some literature research on artificial blood."

"And?"

"It seems to them, and to me, that there are some real questions of legal exposure. Both of the sawbones feel the boy died of injuries that were essentially treatable. They told me that the boy was rocky but that his blood pressure a few minutes before he died was coming back to normal. And it was about that time that Kirk used his artificial blood. The records also show that shortly after he was transfused with the artificial blood, the boy went into cardiac arrest. Both doctors feel there is a possibility that he had an antigen-antibody reaction to the blood product. They would be willing to serve as expert witnesses if this should come to trial."

"All right. But what if all that doesn't hold? You've got a hell of a lot of ifs in there, you know. I don't want Kirk beating a suit and coming out smelling like a hero."

"Oh, hell. Kirk is vulnerable on a dozen things. Even if the blood did not kill the kid directly or prevent him from living long enough so that a surgeon could have a crack at him, I find no evidence that Kirk talked about the use of the blood with his family. He used a product not yet approved for human experimentation on that boy without even discussing it with his parents, much less asking for or getting specific consent. He's left himself wide open to a malpractice complaint. Not just against him, by the way. We, or shall I say his parents, can sue the University as well, even though the kid did not die there. The University, after all, has ultimate responsibility for the research project."

"Okay, I'm convinced. How do we get the family involved? You can't solicit a lawsuit."

"As the attorney for the hospital, after hearing what my experts had to say about all of this, I felt justified to pursue the investigation further. I saw the boy's family."

"Are you nuts?"

"I was careful, Al. I know how to handle these things. I sent one of my investigators to see them. He told them more information was needed about their son, their experience at the hospital. In the course of asking questions, he just happened to mention my name and put some doubts in their minds. Sure enough, they came to see me. Was everything possible done for the son, they wanted to know. Very carefully, mind you, I hinted that even more than necessary was done. I asked, had they signed any consent forms authorizing any type of experimental procedure? It took a while but they got the picture." He stopped when he noticed Anthony's agitated expression. "What's wrong with you?"

"Good lord, Harrison. Why did you go off half-cocked like that? I just wanted a preliminary feeling whether we had anything on Kirk or not. Didn't it ever cross your mind that if you put the idea of a lawsuit in their heads, that they would sue Coit Hill as well?"

"I should take that as a personal offense, Al. Of course it occurred to me. What kind of an idiot do you take me for? I laid it all out for them. Who Kirk was, what his relationship to Coit Hill is. What his relationship to the University is. They came to understand they had little to gain by suing us. I explained to them that they already had enough potential defendants with enough resources to sue and that even if they were able to squeeze a couple of hundred thousand dollars out of us in a settlement that would be peanuts compared to what they could get by having us on their side. Especially since any settlement they got out of us would be diminished by the third or half that would go to their lawyers."

Anthony had half risen out of his chair. "And they bought that? You don't think they'd opt anyway for another two hundred thou, lawyer fees or not?"

"Sit down and let me finish. I indicated that in exchange for a release of liability on the part of the hospital, the hospital would consent to have its attorney—me—represent them in the suit against Kirk and the University. At no cost to them."

"That was generous of you."

"Not quite. They won't be paying, but Coit Hill will. And you'd better figure on about one hundred and fifty thousand dollars."

"I was sure that if anyone made out in this deal, it would be you."

"What I'm doing for you would be a bargain at twice the price." Cummings glanced at his watch. "I've got to get to the office. If you want to talk some more, come upstairs while I get dressed."

Anthony followed the lawyer up the spiral staircase to the second floor and into Cummings's bedroom. One wall was an expanse of glass giving onto the Pacific. The room was carpeted in a deep-pile salmon-colored rug. There was a king-size water bed and two end tables, each buried under books, but no other furniture. A sunken marble jacuzzi, set in a cedar wood deck, graced one corner of the bedroom. Beyond it, Anthony could see a bathroom tiled in pink. A walk-in closet (the size of his own office, Anthony reflected) held all of Cummings's clothes. One wall-length rack held his slacks, another was divided between sport coats and suits. There were shelves and shelves of shirts and sweaters.

Cummings threw off his robe and walked into the closet. Anthony looked around for a place to sit down, considered the water bed, decided against it, and finally deposited himself on the edge of the jacuzzi deck. Cummings, in pants and shirt, came out of the closet.

"Well? What do you think of my little plan?"

"Basically it's okay, but I'm not sure it goes far enough."

"All of a sudden it doesn't go far enough?"

"No. I think the lawsuit will shake Kirk up, all right. But I don't think it will stop him. I know how these things go. You get handed the court papers showing that a lawsuit has been filed against you and you think the world has come to an end. But then the whole thing is turned over to a lawyer. That whole bullshit and rigmarole of depositions, demurrers, continuances starts and, pretty soon, somehow the whole thing loses its threat. The lawsuit becomes the lawyer's problem and for you it becomes just one more nuisance in your life."

"So you'd rather not sue at all?"

"I didn't say that. I think we're going to have to put on more heat if we are going to get to Kirk and really make him a liability to the University."

Cummings walked back into the closet and came out knotting a tie. "What, then, would you do?"

"Two things. Inform the National Institutes of Health about Kirk's little experiment with our patient and see to it that they stop funding Kirk's research. That won't mean the end to the possibility that artificial blood will come along because there's a University of Chicago group pursuing the same lines of research Kirk is. Hell, there's even a couple of private companies experimenting with recombinant DNA techniques to make blood components with chemicals off the shelf. So it's not as if we're setting medical science back one hundred years by taking a whack at Kirk. Beyond informing NIH, I say we should file a complaint with the Board of Medical Quality Assurance and go after Kirk's medical license."

Cummings, rooted in the middle of the room, stared at Anthony with unabashed astonishment. "Don't you think that is going a bit far? After all, you don't have to destroy the guy. You just want him out of your way."

Anthony stood up. "There is only one way to deal with someone like that and it is to do the job right, Cummings. Otherwise he'll just come back to haunt you."

Allan parked his car, locked it, and began walking toward the emergency-room doors, the route he customarily took to gain access to the hospital. But halfway through the parking lot he stopped. In a telephone conversation Fedder had told him that Younger's most recent article, under a headline prominently displaying the words "Mandate for Carnage," had been posted on a bulletin board in the physicians' lounge. While the reaction to him after the first Younger article had been merely chilly, this time around his greeting in the hospital would probably be out-and-out hostility. He bent his head, closed his eyes, and tried to visualize the route that would take him to the jogger's bedside quickly, yet expose him to the smallest possible number of nurses and physicians. After a moment, he headed to the main entrance to the hospital. Few of the University's professional people would be found in the large lobby there. And the stairs off to one side would take him almost directly into the intensive-care unit.

The jogger lay naked on his bed, save for the wrinkled and stained sheet someone had tossed across the lower part of his abdomen. Joe Santorre, Maggie Brooks, two residents new to the trauma service, two interns, and a trauma specialist visiting the University from Baltimore were crowded around the X-ray view boxes near his bed, studying the eight X rays on them. Allan joined them, exchanged light greetings, then stepped in front of his colleagues to study the films. He concentrated on two, one in the upper left-hand corner that had been taken eight days earlier and showed clear and healthy lungs and the latest, tucked into the lower right-hand corner of the box, which was almost completely opaque.

He spoke up: "Summary, Dr. Brooks?"

"This thirty-two-year-old white male was jogging across a street when he was hit broadside by an automobile. He sustained epidural hemorrhage, bilateral rib fractures, bilateral hemopneumothoraces, extensive abdominal injuries including a major tear of the hepatic vein as it attaches to the inferior vena cava, shattered spleen, and multiple traumatic tears of the small and large bowel, extensive retroperitoneal bleeding, a crushed pelvis, tib-fib fracture of the right, and femoral fracture on the left. He also sustained multiple contusions and abrasions.

"The epidural hemorrhage was evacuated, the intra-abdominal bleeding was controlled, splenectomy was performed, fractures were splinted, and he was maintained on the ventilator. He was transfused thirty-seven units of blood. Postoperatively he developed severe clotting abnormalities and required reexploration with extensive packing of the retroperitoneum. Following the second procedure, he stabilized. His bleeding parameters returned to normal. He was maintained on the ventilator. He developed progressive deterioration of renal function and was started on dialysis. On his third postinjury day, he was returned to the operating room for removal of packs. This was done without complication.

"Until forty-eight hours ago, it appeared as though he was making progress. His renal function was showing improvement with return of urine output and progressive improvement in his breathing status. For the past two days he has been spiking temperatures as high as one hundred and four. Blood cultures were positive for pseudomonas. His renal function has deteriorated. He has developed signs of liver failure and his pulmonary function has deteriorated. Extensive workup for the cause of the pseudomonas infection has been unrewarding to date. All IV lines have been changed. He has been bronchoscoped with no clarification of the problem. Plain X rays of the abdomen have been negative as has been an ultrasound. CAT scan of the abdomen is pending."

And with that Maggie, who had not consulted any notes, finished her unemotional, laconic review of the jogger's condition.

Allan nodded. "Thank you, Dr. Brooks." Moving to the jogger's side, he lifted the chart from the hook by which it hung at the end of the bed and thumbed through the scores of pages within it. He scrutinized temperatures, lab results. He stepped back to the X rays, studied them again, then returned to the jogger's side. Each time Allan moved, the residents and interns moved, like sandpipers moving back and forth with a running tide.

Gently, he checked the jogger's skin, studied the veins in the neck, drew back the eyelids and studied the whites and the pupils of the eyes. Lightly, he ran his hand down the jogger's chest, pressed against the abdomen.

"Well, doctor," he said, addressing Maggie. "You've told us that we have evidence of an infection and that we have not been able to localize it. Any further ideas?"

"Although the workup has not shown the source, we know he's septic and the most likely source is the abdominal cavity. We should explore. But I'm afraid he would not tolerate a major operation."

"You're on the right track," Allan said, then turned to Santorre. "Get a CAT scan on him and set him up for six units of blood. Let's wait to see what the scan shows. But if it doesn't localize the site of infection, then we have no choice but to go in. Brooks, come with me to talk to his wife. She should be aware of what we are doing, that his chances of making it are very small, but that an operation is our only chance. We're going to have to tell her that he could die on the table."

Maggie's jaw tightened, but she nodded and followed Allan out of the room, toward the visitors' lounge where the jogger's wife was waiting. As they passed the nurses' station on their way out of the intensive-care unit, a nurse signaled to Allan that he had a telephone call.

"Tell 'em I'll call them back," he said, hurrying past.

"It's Dr. Dorr's secretary. She says it's urgent."

With a resigned slouching of the shoulders, he stopped and turned to Maggie. "Do me a favor? Talk to the wife by yourself."

"Allan!" There was desperation in her voice. "Not for this. I can't go out there and tell her her husband needs an operation that could kill him."

"Maggie, if she can take the news from anyone, she can take it from you. I hear you've built up a tremendous relationship with her. You don't have to tell her her husband will die. Hold it out as a possibility. Just as it is a possibility that we can pull him through and solve this latest setback. Go on."

He watched her push dejectedly through the double doors, then turned to answer the phone.

"I'm sorry to disturb you, Dr. Kirk," Dorr's secretary said, "but there is an urgent letter for you here. May I bring it down to you?"

"I'm in the middle of rounds. It'll keep. I'll get it later."

"I think I had best bring it down to you, doctor. I'll be there in a minute."

Annoyed and apprehensive, he walked to the nearby bank of elevators. One of the doors opened and Dorr's secretary started to rush out, but stopped when she saw him, holding the door open with one hand while she motioned to him with the envelope she held in her other hand. "Dr. Dorr said to tell you it would be best if you opened this in private," she said, handing him the envelope. "I'm sorry, the phones are unattended and I have to get back." With that she released the button, the doors slammed shut, and she was gone.

Allan stared at the envelope. The return address belonged to a law firm in town. He frowned, puzzled as to why a letter from a law firm would have Dorr and his secretary in such an uproar. At least once a month one of the trauma victims who'd been brought to the hospital would die and become the centerpiece of a homicide or vehicular-manslaughter case; then Allan would have to give a deposition so that the county's prosecuting attorney could proceed with a case against the alleged killer or reckless driver. Why the excitement now? he wondered.

He wandered into the surgical lounge to read the letter. He stuffed the envelope into a back pocket and poured himself his traditional cup of coffee well fortified with four heaping teaspoons of sugar. Sipping, he scanned the letter quickly, expecting to find the usual convoluted phraseology asking his pardon for impinging on his time, but nevertheless going on to tell him that his expert testimony would be needed in a prosecution. But the familiar wording was not there. The letter was telling him that he would be named in a malpractice lawsuit, that he was being held responsible for the death of one Greg Gerbetti who had died while under his care in the emergency room of Coit Hill Memorial Medical Center. Said death, the letter read, had been due to his general negligence, his inability to make a proper and timely diagnosis, his negligence in providing proper care, and his willful use of a medication not approved for human experimentation.

He read the letter again. Feelings and thoughts left him, then came rushing back, tripping over each other in a jumble of questions tinged by fear. His heart was beating rapidly, a sensation rapidly displaced by an urge to run to the bathroom. The last time he had willfully had to fight that urge was when he had gone to tell his father that he would be specializing in trauma medicine.

Questions ramrodded through his head. What the hell are they talking about? Negligence? I busted my butt trying to keep that kid alive until we could get someone in to take him to surgery. *Was* it the artificial blood that killed him? Had there been an adverse reaction to it? What else could I have done? Negligence? The whole damned system is negligent. That boy and I got caught up in it. If they are suing me, are they also suing Coit Hill? Or any of the physicians whose names appeared on the emergency-room chart, followed by the notation, "Called but unavailable"?

Dorr was right, Allan said to himself: I crossed Anthony and now I am going to pay. He shuffled to the in-house telephone and dialed Dorr's number; Dorr was tied up in an emergency meeting but had left instructions for Allan to come to his house that evening, promptly at eight.

The private phone in Anthony's office chimed softly. Anthony, who had been staring out the window, a self-satisfied grin on his face, answered it to find Cummings on the other end.

"The letter was hand delivered this morning, Al. We're on our way."

"Good. Now, do you know what else you can do?"

"I shudder to think," Cummings answered, responding to the lilt of satisfaction in Anthony's voice.

"Have someone at your office call the *Mirror* and leak the

letter and the lawsuit against Kirk and the University.

"Why the *Mirror*? Why not Younger at the *Telegraph*?"

"Because Kirk is quite obviously Younger's hero at the moment. Younger would use the story—he couldn't afford not to—but he'd wind up linking the suit to the hearing the other night, or to me."

Cummings laughed. "You mean he'd write a balanced story and put it all in context. Why wouldn't the *Mirror* do the same thing?"

"Maybe they would, but I doubt it. They're coming into this late so they don't have Younger's background. Oh, they'll call Kirk and the hospital and the parents for comments. But I would bet that the instinct would be to use the story to show that the competition's fair-haired boy is not quite the Dr. Schweitzer the *Telegraph* would have us believe."

Dorr, dressed in old jeans and a sweatshirt and holding a drink, let Allan in and guided him to the living room.

"Would you like something to drink? I have some soda or juice, if you'd like." Dorr was trying to be friendly, casual, but Allan didn't miss the obligatory tone of the offer. He asked for orange juice, then took a seat while Dorr went off to the kitchen.

"I guess I really don't know what to say, Phil," Allan said when Dorr returned with his drink.

Dorr put down his glass and sat down. "Why did you do it, Allan? How could you possibly take an experimental product like that and not only use it without authorization on a patient, but use it in an institution where you shouldn't even have been working in the first place? What the hell were you doing at Coit Hill, anyway? Why did you even have it with you?"

"I was at Coit Hill because I've been trying to make some extra money to pay off some loans, Phil. I had packets of the blood with me because it occurred to me that we were testing everything about the blood except its sensitivity to transportation. There was no reason why carting it around in an ambulance bouncing over city streets would render it unstable, for example, but I wanted to be sure. Every time I came back to the hospital, I would take some out of my trunk and test it."

"And?"

"It always tested out all right. I was going to bring the rest of the batch in that morning anyway. If I had worked at Coit Hill the following evening, I would not have had the artificial blood with me."

"Well, that still doesn't answer the main question. Whatever possessed you to use it?"

"I never would have used it if we were just beginning to work with the blood or if it hadn't been tested. I used it because I didn't have a choice. That boy was dying on me. I couldn't get anyone to come in to operate. I took a chance and I blew it. But, apart from this set-up lawsuit, I'm not sorry I tried. Under the circumstances, it was reasonable to do so. The next step is using it on humans anyway."

"Yes, but under controlled conditions. And more important, with approval from the FDA and informed consent from the patients. Good lord, you know that when we use anything experimental at the University we have the patient sign a form that's as long as his discharge bill."

"What kind of consent am I supposed to get from a near-corpse?"

"The family was there."

"It would have taken me twenty minutes just to explain all the pros and cons and indications and counterindications. It was an extreme situation and I used extreme methods."

"So you did. And now we are all reaping the consequences."

"What do you mean, 'we'?"

"Allan, the University is being sued as well because we're helping sponsor your research. Not only that, but word is out about your using the blood and about the lawsuit by the Gerbetti family. Not half an hour ago I got a call from the *Mirror*, wanting to know about the artificial blood and how many people we've used it on. I can guarantee you that within twenty-four hours after that story hits the streets, every family who has had someone die after being treated at the University after an accident will find an attorney and all those shysters will be fishing for the same thing. They'll be convinced that the people who died received the artificial blood and that they have grounds for suing the University."

"Phil . . ."

"Let me finish. You work hard and you're dedicated. You've got charisma. If you were in private practice you'd have to turn patients away or work twenty-four hours a day. If you were to stay in academia, you could head your own surgical department in no time . . . except for your impulsive way of doing things. Who said you suddenly had to go off and lead a fight for a trauma center?"

"I'm not leading a fight for anything," Allan started to protest.

"Yes, you are. Now that you sounded off before the Joint Committee for Emergency Services, you are."

"That's not fair, Phil. I didn't say anything we haven't said around the lunch table for years now."

"Talking about deficits in trauma services over a sandwich in the cafeteria is not the same as airing the subject in public, Allan, and you know it. You've stirred up the medical community, and especially the community hospitals who feel threatened by the slightest thing that might change patient referral patterns. Worse yet, you've taken on Anthony. You've played right into the hands of our own administrator, who, as you know, is not overly fond of you, and into the hands of people who are still angry about the decision to establish the trauma service."

"I'm sorry they all see it so negatively."

"You should not have expected anything else. I was tied up in meetings all day because of you. One of the meetings was of the hospital board, a special meeting called at the behest of the administrator."

Allan watched his mentor. The older man met his glance for a second, looked down at his feet, then looked back up. Allan sank back in his chair.

"I'm sorry, but the board has decided to withdraw your appointment as head of the trauma department. I'm asking you now to take a leave from the surgical department. I think I should warn you, though, that there is also very serious talk about having you resign completely from the University. In fact, it is more than likely that the request for you to do so will be forthcoming shortly."

"Phil . . . ," Allan began to plead.

"Allan. I tried to warn you. There was nothing I could do. When you make enemies the way you have, you can't expect mercy when they finally have you up against the wall. I know it sounds bad and I can't kid you—careers have been ruined under similar circumstances. But I think you could still have a future, if you make yourself invisible for a while. Concentrate on the lab work in the meantime. The University has competent legal counsel and, of course, they'll handle your case. But until things are settled and have quieted down, keep out of the way. In fact, if I were you, I would even get out of town for a few days. It'll lessen the temptation to do something foolish."

When Cummings phoned Anthony to tell him the news, he could almost visualize the look of ecstasy on the other man's face. No fewer than five people—one parent, two wives, one husband, and one "spouse equivalent"—had called to tell the attorney that, having seen the article about Allan in the *Mirror*, they wanted to retain his firm to represent them in suits against Allan and the University.

"You going to do it?" Anthony asked.

"Of course, what do you think? In fact, we're going to make a kind of a legal Chinese water torture out of this. I'm going to take those cases and file them one a day over a period of one week. By the time the last suit is filed on a Friday, both the University and Kirk will be ready to close up shop."

9

Anthony, working to keep an encouraging and warm smile on his face, watched as the mayor and the San Francisco county supervisor for the district in which Coit Hill was located strapped themselves into their seats in the helicopter.

"It's your dog-and-pony show, Al," the supervisor said, leaning forward in his seat so he could look out the narrow door. "You sure you can't come along and give us your personal rebuttal to Kirk's contentions that you don't need this hunk of tin?"

"George, this is not meant as a rebuttal to anything or anyone," Anthony answered. "We just thought it would be nice to have you and the mayor out and show you what kind of service we are giving your district and the city. Anyway, I've got a working dinner I arranged before this came up and I can't get out of it. Enjoy the ride."

Anthony stepped back to the edge of the concrete pad and watched as the giant rotor blade slowly began to make its sweeping circles through the air. When the craft finally lifted up, Anthony waved, then turned and trotted back to the side door leading into the hospital. He stopped again and turned to study the pad, then made a mental note to get the maintenance department finally to paint on it the Coit Hill Memorial Medical Center sign he had ordered weeks earlier. The giant yellow and red letters, he thought, would look marvelous from high in the sky.

The pilot, who had concentrated on lifting the helicopter well above the hospital, turned to his passengers. "Gentlemen," he shouted to be heard above the din, "to start off, let's assume that we've had a call from the naval base over on Yerba Buena Island. We're going to treat this run as if we were flying out, picking up a trauma victim to get him back here."

"Would you get such a call?" the supervisor yelled back. "Wouldn't the Navy be able to take care of their own problems out there?"

"Might in most cases. But in a case of real trauma, sure they'd call us. I'm going to radio ahead to the base to tell 'em we're coming. No sense surprising the military. Supervisor Page, why don't you time our run?"

Page looked at his watch to note the time, then pressed his forehead against the door window to watch the city sweep by beneath them. The Civic Center, with its new Opera House, its stately government buildings, popped into view, then disappeared. Market Street, the freeway, the docks of the Embarcadero swept by beneath them. They streaked just above and to the right of the San Francisco–Oakland Bay Bridge and within moments the choppy waters of the Bay gave way to the brown and barren terrain of Yerba Buena Island.

"Time?" the pilot called out.

The supervisor looked at his watch. "Seven minutes, twenty seconds."

"Add a minute or so to touch down, maybe five minutes to pick up the victim, and another three minutes to get back, and you see that even if a trauma patient is in a difficult-to-reach place like this one we could have him back at Coit Hill in about sixteen minutes of receiving a call."

"How about if someone is hurt at, say, Candlestick? What would be the timing of that?" the mayor asked.

"Good question. Let's take a swing over and see." The pilot lifted the helicopter higher into the air, guided it through a sweeping turn toward the south, then flew along the edge of the city, passed over Hunter's Point, and, lowering the chopper, hovered over the stadium.

"Looks like the Giants have a workout going. Crappy way they're playing, they sure need it," he shouted. "Mayor, let's say a lady has been hit in the chest by a line-drive foul and we've just picked her up after landing in that parking lot over to the right. Supervisor, start timing us."

With a sharp jerk, the helicopter veered off to the left. McClaren Park, Twin Peaks, Seventeenth Street, the Panhandle to Golden Gate Park rolled by. "We're above the hospital," the pilot called out. "What was our time?"

"Eight minutes, thirty seconds," Page answered. "Very impressive. But that was the easy stuff." He looked down as the helicopter described a wide circle around the crowded area where Coit Hill was located. "What about a call for someone who's lying in a busy street?"

"All right," the pilot called back. "Let's look for a crowded situation."

They cruised the central city's residential and commercial neighborhoods until the mayor spotted an intersection where traffic had come to a standstill. Cars and buses stood immobile in every direction on the two narrow streets.

"Let's say that someone was hurt down there in that white Oldsmobile," the mayor said. "Where in the world would you put down?"

The pilot craned his neck, first to look for the car the mayor had singled out, then to survey the urban sprawl beneath them. "There is always somewhere you can put down," he answered. "A rooftop, another intersection a block away, a vacant lot. Even a playground like that one half a block from the Olds. Let's put in there and show you."

"In the middle of all those power and telephone lines?" the mayor asked, looking down on the wires crisscrossing near the area the pilot had designated.

"No sweat. Flying around those like a pigeon is the first maneuver they teach us. Start your watch, supervisor."

Feeling the craft begin to lower, Page pushed the buttons that brought the timing display on his watch to 0:00.00. But in the sudden lurching and shuddering that followed he realized that something was wrong. He forgot his role as timekeeper of the practice rescue run and instead gripped the armrests of his seat.

Everett Huntington leaned back in his chair, threw his feet up on the corner of the desk, and rested his coffee mug on his stomach. For the first time since the office was finished two days earlier, he had time to sit down and savor the new surroundings Anthony had promised and built for him. Light-years away from what he had had at the University. Instead of a government-issued steel desk, he was blessed with a smart walnut worktable that rested on two modern-design filing cabinets. The wall to his left was covered by new bookshelves holding dozens of brand-new reference books and, in newly bound volumes, also courtesy of Anthony, all the journals he considered crucial to his efforts to keep up to date with emergency medicine trends. At the University, on those nights he could not go home he often had had to sleep on a small lumpy cot in a room shared, all too often, with residents and interns. Here, just beyond the bookshelves, a door opened into his private sleeping quarters. The single bed was ample and comfortable. There was a nightstand, a radio/alarm clock, a twelve-inch color television, and a small refrigerator one of the dietitians kept well stocked. He even had his own bathroom, complete with a shower that doubled as a mini-steamroom.

Huntington looked through the wall-to-ceiling plate-glass sheet that separated his office from the emergency room. His eyes shone with affection and satisfaction. Finally, he had his own domain. At the University, Allan Kirk, Joe Santorre, and the other trauma surgeons had always been in his hair, demanding to take immediate charge of the patients, overriding his decisions to have tests performed, pooh-poohing other tests he insisted on having. There had never been a day when he hadn't been involved in disagreements with Allan and his bunch, when conflicts between him and the trauma people had not been part and parcel of the response to patients. But this was his kingdom. He was running the emergency room. He, not some trauma wise guy, was seeing patients first, deciding what to do with them, which tests to order, what consultants to call in.

And yet consultants, Huntington sighed, were also the thorn in his side here. He had often wished that Allan and the other egomaniacs at the University did not insist on getting in his way as often as they did, but he couldn't argue with the fact that they knew what they were doing when faced with somebody who'd been turned into raw hamburger in a freeway crunch. Egos notwithstanding, at Coit Hill there was no one who approached their abilities. Anthony had tried to hire two or three young trauma surgeons. But each one had turned him down, apparently because rumors had reached them of Anthony's dictatorial dealings with the hospital's anesthesiologists and radiologists. So when he needed to call in surgeons to deal with a trauma patient, he still had to depend on old-time general surgeons who loved to treat him to rambling lectures on how a gallbladder problem or a hernia was a "trauma" every bit as serious as a crushed spleen. What a bunch of dumb old farts, he said to himself.

With a jerk he threw his feet off the desk and reached for the coffeepot standing on the small table near his chair. But the motion was interrupted by a crackling on the intercom. "Dr. Huntington," Cluny's voice called out to him. "There's been a major accident apparently involving the mayor and Supervisor Page."

Huntington leaned forward to press the talk button. "They were supposed to be in our chopper getting a firsthand demonstration."

"The helicopter crashed, doctor. An ambulance is bringing the mayor and the pilot in here. According to the paramedics, their injuries aren't all that bad."

"And Page?"

"He sustained more serious injuries. He was triaged to the University."

Huntington stood and hurried to the front desk. Cluny, her face expressionless, her hands clasped together in front of her, was waiting for him. Damned bitch, Huntington said to himself, she's been around so long she probably treated Eve for snakebite, but she still stands there like a private waiting for her marching orders even though she knows very well what has to be done.

"Miss Cluny," he said slowly, trying to put some sweetness

into his voice. Despite his feelings, he knew her reputation and didn't want to offend her. "Please call the O.R. and tell them to have a crew stand by. And oh, yes, one more thing. Would you mind checking the on-call list and letting me know what surgeons can be reached."

Cluny turned on her heels and disappeared. A minute later she was back. "Drs. Dayton, Okatani, and Adams are on call, doctor," she informed him. "Should I call them after I've taken care of the other matters?"

He counted to five. "No, that's all right," he said. "I'll call them myself."

He found the list of doctors' phone numbers and ran his finger down the names until he reached Dr. Dayton's. Automatically, he glanced at his watch. It was 6:30. Please, God, he said in silent prayer as he now picked up the telephone, I know Dayton lives in San Rafael and that it takes him a good hour to get home. But please let today be the one day he left the hospital early.

Dr. Dayton's wife told Huntington that Dayton had not left the hospital until 5:45. Slowly Huntington put down the phone. He knew Dayton would be sitting in the middle of bumper-to-bumper traffic on the Golden Gate Bridge. Even if I beeped him now, Huntington told himself, he wouldn't get to a phone for another thirty minutes. It would be at least another hour before he had managed to turn around and return to the hospital.

"You don't have to bother calling Dr. Okatani, either," Cluny's cold and precise voice informed him. "He lives in Redwood City."

"San Rafael and Redwood City. Terrific. Why are these people on the on-call list?"

"Because they were willing to commit to handling trauma patients, Dr. Huntington. They understand what is at stake, I imagine."

"I guess I'll try Adams. He does live fairly close, if I remember."

Huntington held the phone in his hand and mulled his decision, wondering if there were someone else he could try. He was not keen to call Adams, a surgeon in his early sixties. The man had been pressured by Anthony into providing trauma coverage.

Knowing his own shortcomings, he usually tried to find one hundred reasons why a trauma patient should not be operated on immediately. And yet, having no choice, Huntington dialed his number. Before the third ring had finished, he could hear the sound of the ambulance siren. He shoved the phone at Cluny with instructions to tell Adams to get himself in to the hospital, called to two orderlies to bring gurneys, summoned the second emergency-room nurse, and ran outside.

While the others lifted the pilot to one of the rolling beds, he helped the ambulance driver and the other paramedic take the mayor out of the vehicle.

"Get their clothes off," Huntington yelled out as they wheeled the two men into the emergency room, "and get X Ray to bring a portable machine down here. Get the lab down here, we're going to have to cross and match blood. Set up IVs and—"

"Young fella." It was the mayor, tugging at Huntington's sleeve. "Take it easy, young man. We're just fine. No sense getting yourself all steamed up. I am having just a little trouble getting my breath and it hurts some when I breathe deeply. But other than that I feel great." Huntington looked down at the mayor. The man had a large face with generous jowls and heavy eyebrows. His mouth seemed to have been etched into a permanent smile and his eyes twinkled as he spoke. "Just take it nice and slow, and everything will be just fine." He lay back down contented.

Huntington, his stride broken, found himself following the mayor's instructions. Working at a slower pace, he checked the IV lines a nurse had placed even as the mayor was giving his little speech, then began to paste the electrocardiogram sensors in place around the mayor's chest. The mayor tugged at his sleeve again. "And, young man, let's keep the EKG results quiet. I had a heart attack about nine months ago, which is not well known. Keep in mind that I'm running for governor and have a state primary coming up soon, will you?" He gave Huntington a broad wink.

Huntington smiled back. He glanced over to the helicopter pilot and saw that Cluny was working on the man, who was also engaged in an animated conversation with her. Assured, Huntington picked up the last EKG sensor and pressed it against the mayor's upper abdomen. Immediately he sensed danger. The mayor's muscles tensed. The politician groaned. "You'd better check that blood pressure again," Huntington said to the nurse who was working with him. He cast his patient a nervous glance. "And let's get a chest film."

"Pressure dropped down to seventy."

A technician rolled the portable X-ray machine to the mayor's bedside. "Send for some blood, hurry up, and set up so we can tap his belly. He must be bleeding. We'd better find out where it's coming from," Huntington ordered, even as he helped place the X-ray equipment over the mayor's chest. The technician took the X ray, then pushed the machine away.

"Ten cc's novocaine, scalpel, and the catheter," Huntington barked. "Come on, come on." Within seconds, he anesthetized the area below the navel, cut an opening into the belly, and inserted the catheter. Blood poured out.

"He's got a belly full of blood." Huntington was sweating now, conscious that Adams had not yet made his appearance in the emergency room.

"Is Adams coming in or not?" he yelled at Cluny.

"He had just gotten home when I called. He said he'd be here as soon as possible."

"As soon as possible? This man should be in the operating room in five minutes. Call the O.R. Tell them we're on our way up. Maybe by the time we get there, Adams will be in. Keep an eye on the pilot. If he starts to sour in any way, call me down. And have the tech send the X ray up to the O.R.!"

They were turning into the operating room when Adams, already in his greens, emerged from the doctor's changing room. "Would anyone mind filling me in on the details?" he asked.

"The mayor was in a helicopter crash," Huntington recounted for him quickly. "He came in looking stable, the only obvious injury being rib fractures bilaterally. But we tapped his belly and he's full of blood."

Adams examined the mayor. "He looks pretty stable to me now. Maybe we'd be better off observing him in the ICU." The surgeon was clearly nervous. "Let's have an internist come in and look at him too."

Huntington, aware that the mayor was looking back and

forth between him and Adams as if watching a television debate, drew Adams aside. "Look, you've got to trust me. I've seen a lot of cases like this. We have to go in. Now!"

Adams spread his hand across the lower half of his face and drew down. The bottom portion of his eyes showed and his mouth twisted out of shape. "All right, all right. Let's go in. The gasser is in already and is changing clothes as well."

To Huntington, the time that elapsed before Adams and the anesthesiologist finally entered the operating room were interminable. "Let's get a move on, fellas," he snapped when they appeared in the door, "before he turns to shit!!"

Working across from Adams as his assistant, Huntington watched the surgeon work in the mayor's abdominal cavity and make a determined effort to trace and stop the bleeding. Huntington began to relax. But then the feeling was shattered by the shrill, insistent buzzing of the electronic blood-pressure machine. In a well-synchronized move, the heads of the three doctors and the three nurses in the operating room snapped toward the small black box elevated just to the right of the patient's shoulder. The digital readout, which, thanks to the infusions of fluids, had shown a comfortable 110/70 at the beginning of the operation, now stood at 60/40.

"What the hell is going on?" Adams asked.

The anesthesiologist glanced at the EKG machine keeping track of the mayor's heart rate. "Not exactly sure," he said. "I've got the IV running wide open. Can you give me some aortic compression?"

"Blood pressure is down to 40/20," Huntington said quietly.

"What the hell is going on?" Adams repeated, looking from Huntington to the anesthesiologist, then back to Huntington again, hoping that someone would tell him what his next step ought to be.

"What's his neck veins look like?" Huntington called to the anesthesiologist.

"Distended."

"Goddamnit," Huntington said. "It must be a pericardial tamponade. Adams, you're going to have to open his chest."

"Crack his chest?" Shaking his head, Adams reached for a

scalpel, then placed it between the mayor's fourth and fifth ribs, and cut through the skin and muscle.

"He's straightlined us," the anesthesiologist called out. "He's arrested."

Adams, acting on reflex, plunged his hand into the chest opening and grabbed the heart.

"What do you feel?" Huntington asked.

"God, I don't know. I can't tell." Adams looked down at his hand, as if wondering how it had gotten into the mayor's chest.

Huntington pushed Adams out of the way, reached into the chest, and squeezed. "Give me a couple of amps of bicarbonate and an amp of epinephrine," he called out.

Keeping his eyes on the EKG monitor, waiting for the drugs to elicit a response, Huntington squeezed and squeezed.

"Huntington, hold off for a second, let me check his rhythm," the anesthesiologist said. "I can't get a proper reading as long as you're doing the work for his heart." Huntington stopped. They turned to the EKG monitor. A flat beige line ran along the green screen. When the line faded as it reached the edge of the monitor, another flat line followed it quickly.

Coit Hill's autopsy room was a study in stainless steel. Drawers, shelves, dissection tables, microscopes, and the instruments arrayed on trays all shone and sparkled with the bluish tint of fluorescent lighting on metal. Harrison Cummings, dressed in a raggedy turtleneck sweater, cotton pants, and torn deck shoes, had taken a chair close to the morgue room door, as far as possible from the single, sheet-covered body. Sherman Harper was at the only desk in the room, his arms folded across his chest, his eyes closed, his mouth slightly open. Anthony, his jaw set, his right hand kneading his right temple, paced back and forth across the clean marble floor, the taps on his heels beating out the cadence of his march. He stopped in front of Cummings.

"Can you believe this? We've got a dead mayor in here. Huntington is nowhere in sight and the frigging pathologist has been holed up in that goddamn cubicle for an hour, like he was studying for his first boards. What the fuck is going on?!"

"Al, calm down," Cummings said. "It's not going to help to have a stroke."

Anthony resumed his pacing, sticking both hands between the small of his back and his pants, looking from time to time first at his watch, then to the locked door behind which the pathologist was studying the results of the hurried autopsy he had performed on the mayor.

Harper slowly opened his eyes and watched the hospital administrator. "Well, Al," he said slowly. "A CAT scanner may be large, gray, and ugly, but it sure as hell doesn't crash with VIPs in it, does it?"

Anthony wheeled. "You're enjoying this, aren't you, Sherman? You're just lapping it up, right?" He stepped closer to his chief of staff and eyed him with unrestrained malevolence.

"No, as a matter of fact, I'm not enjoying this at all. I can well imagine what the fallout is going to be."

"There won't be any fallout, Sherman. None at all."

Harper turned. "We've lost a half-million-dollar helicopter. The mayor of this city, the man everyone was betting to be the next governor of the state, dies in our operating room. And you say there won't be consequences?"

"None. The chopper crashed because the asshole who was flying it didn't know what he was doing. The bastard lied to us about his experience. It was unfortunate, but it happens. We'll just be more stringent in checking out the next guy we hire, that's all."

"Al, you're joking. The next guy we hire? You're going to buy another helicopter?"

"Why the hell not? In fact, Sherman, I'm going to buy not one, but two."

Even Cummings could not repress what sounded like a snort.

"What the hell is so funny? The insurance will replace the one that went down. We'll find the money for the second one. This just proves what I've suspected all along, that we need a second, backup helicopter. And, goddamnit, we're going to get it. I'm going to pick—"

Anthony's sentence hung unfinished as the door to the morgue opened and Huntington stepped in to the room. He was still in the surgical greens he had worn during the operation on the mayor some five hours earlier.

"It's about goddamn time," Anthony said between compressed lips. "Where the hell have you been?"

Huntington shrugged. "We had a pileup on the freeway. We got six people in with minor lacerations and first- and second-degree burns. We got those squared away but the driver of one of the cars had seizures and we couldn't get them under control. I couldn't get away."

"All right, never mind," Anthony said. "Want to give us your rundown on what happened?"

"We had an aggressive resuscitative effort. I think everyone did well. The nursing staff, the surgeon, the anesthesiologist. It was all going like clockwork. We had the mayor in the O.R. fast, had the abdomen open, and the source of the bleeding identified. Then it all went to hell. He arrested on us."

"We know all that, doctor," Cummings said. "But why did he arrest?"

"We have a suspicion. When we still had the mayor in the E.R. he acknowledged a history of heart disease, said he had recently had a myocardial infarction. The EKG did show evidence of an old myocardial infarction as well as some acute ischemic changes. As far as I am concerned, I'm comfortable with what happened. Putting it all together, I'd say it was an inevitable death. We just can't save everybody. What's the path report show?"

"It would be nice to know. But Wolfson has been locked in there for an hour and won't come out, or so he said, until he has pieced the whole story together."

"Seeing that he sometimes acts as a deputy coroner, I guess he'd want to take his time," Cummings muttered.

As if on cue the door to the cubicle opened and a tall, angular man walked out. Thin hair, cut short, fell across his forehead. He brushed it back onto his head as he closed the door and faced the group. Anthony, Huntington, Harper, and Cummings watched him as he walked to the covered body.

"Well, Wolfson?" Anthony said.

Wolfson opened the folder he had brought in, took a pair of half-glasses from a pocket in his trousers, and slipped them on. "As you know, we have a case of a sixty-two-year-old white male who was involved in a helicopter accident and sustained multi-system trauma—"

"Will you please cut the bullshit, Wolfson," Anthony grumbled. "We know who and what was involved. Huntington is convinced heart disease killed him. Do you agree or not?"

Wolfson put down the folder and took off his glasses. "Heart disease had nothing to do with this, in my opinion," he said, casting a long glance at Huntington. "The cause of death was cardiac arrest, secondary to a tension pneumothorax."

No one spoke. Cummings, looking at Anthony and the three physicians around the administrator, knew immediately that the silence was one of shock. He took a legal pad and a pen out of the small briefcase he had with him and began to make a list of the work he would have to do in less than eight hours.

"I don't believe it," Anthony said. "What are you talking about?"

Wolfson looked at Anthony, trying to determine if the administrator was really surprised by the information or whether he was trying to imply that the pathologist was fabricating his analysis. He decided Anthony was truly taken aback. "A fractured rib lacerated the lung, in effect producing a one-way valve," Wolfson said, turning his gaze on the rest of the group. "When the anesthesiologist started blowing air into the mayor's lungs under pressure to ventilate him, this converted a rather trivial tear in the lung into a potentially lethal problem. As he pumped more and more air into the lungs, more and more air escaped through the tear into the right chest cavity. Under the pressure of the air in the cavity, the right lung collapsed and pushed the heart and the great vessels over to the left. That stopped the return of blood to the heart."

Cummings was scribbling furiously. "No need to write all this down, Mr. Cummings," Wolfson said. "This will all be in my report. I think you'd be better off for now just listening to what I am saying."

Abashed, Cummings pushed away the pad. "In any case,"

Wolfson continued, "it was a combination of the lack of blood returning to the heart and the collapse of the right lung that led to the cardiac arrest. But it was that combination and not atherosclerotic ischemia that was directly responsible for the death."

"Now let me get something straight," Anthony cut in. "The mayor—"

"There is nothing to get straight, Al," Huntington said in a voice so low the rest had to lean forward to hear what he was saying. "We blew it. We missed a pneumothorax and killed the mayor. He should not have died."

Anthony leaped out of his chair. "Are you out of your mind? What the hell are you talking about? We killed the mayor?"

The pathologist held up his hand. "I don't want to categorize things in terms of who or what killed whom. However, I must say that anyone looking at this autopsy will come to an essentially simple conclusion."

"Which is?" Cummings cut in.

"That a simple chest tube in the right chest would have relieved the pneumothorax."

"God almighty!" Huntington said, burying his face in his hands.

Wolfson looked at him, a search for Huntington's motivations again evident in his eyes. "But that is not to say," the pathologist continued, "that the mayor would have lived. We have to understand, gentlemen, that he was a sixty-two-year-old man, and I did find evidence of underlying heart disease. Perhaps even if the chest tube had been inserted he might still not have been able to survive the stress of the surgery because of his cardiac condition. But I must stress this: there is no question that the diagnosis of a tension pneumothorax was missed, and that had that been treated appropriately he at least would have had a reasonable chance of making it."

Harper, who had said nothing, made no effort to hide his contempt for Huntington. "You had a chest X ray taken, didn't you, Everett?" he sneered at the hapless emergency-room doctor.

"Yes."

"And it never occurred to you to look at it, to look for signs of a possible pneumothorax?"

"I would have looked at it, yes. But when his blood pressure dropped so suddenly, the only thing that occurred to me was to rush him to surgery and hope that Dr. Adams would get there in time to operate."

Harper's face had taken on a prosecutorial demeanor. "Let's be frank here. Adams is not a highly trained trauma surgeon, is he, Everett?"

Huntington shook his head.

"But you were in the operating room and you know as much about trauma as anyone in this hospital. Did it not occur to you to suggest to him to look for further injuries in the chest cavity?"

"I never had time to consider it. Between the time Adams began to go into the abdomen and the moment the mayor went into cardiac arrest, maybe, well, three minutes passed. And that includes the time we took to control the bleeding from the spleen. If he had lived longer, I don't know, I guess I might have suggested that Adams look at the lungs. But I never had a chance to do it."

Harper glanced at Anthony. The mask was gone. The administrator's face was pasty and lined. Anthony closed his eyes and shook his head. No one said a word.

It was Cummings who finally spoke up. "What's the bottom line on this, then?"

"The bottom line, counselor," Harper said in measured words, "is that Huntington is right. The team blew the resuscitation. We killed the mayor. Pure and simple."

The physician's verdict seemed to galvanize Anthony. "Now wait," he said, bolting up in his chair, "who are you to be judge and jury on this?"

"Al, it is patently obvious."

"Nothing is patently obvious." Anthony turned to the pathologist, who was holding all of the records that had been gathered on the mayor. "What was the time of admission?"

The pathologist opened the folder and scanned the first two papers in the file. "Ah, six thirty-seven."

"And what time was he taken to the operating room?"

The pathologist shuffled more papers. "Let's see. Six fifty-two."

"Fifteen minutes from admission to operating table," Anthony trumpeted. "Who's going to argue with that? That's as fast as any trauma service is going to get someone into the operating room. In the operating room, the surgeon found overwhelming injuries incompatible with survival, that's all."

A heavy silence descended on the room. Cummings stared at his hands. The pathologist made a show of leafing through the mayor's files. Huntington leaned back and looked at the ceiling.

Harper spoke next. His voice was hoarse. "You can't just gloss over it like that, Al. It won't wash."

"What am I glossing over, Dr. Harper?" Anthony's voice had taken on a combative note. "What am I glossing over?"

"That a major injury was overlooked."

"Nonsense. The man was in the emergency room for fifteen minutes. In that time, IVs were placed, blood was started, an X ray was taken, and he was rushed to an operating room where a trained surgeon and an anesthesiologist were present. How much more can you do in a quarter of an hour?"

"Just enough to discern another major and obvious injury," Harper persisted quietly.

Anthony was now on his feet. His face shone with self-righteous indignation. "What are you trying to do here, Harper? What do you suggest we do? Hold a press conference at which we turn Drs. Huntington and Adams over to whatever assistant district attorney handles criminal medical cases in this county?"

"Well, n-no," Harper stammered.

"Then again I ask you, what do you suggest we do?" Anthony turned to the rest of the group. "Does anyone here have any other bright ideas?"

Huntington stood and paced the room. He glanced at the mayor's covered body, then turned back to face his colleagues. "Al, what are you trying to do?" he asked. "It's one thing to make an error in treatment. I'm willing to own up to that. It's another thing to try to distort the facts. I'm sorry, I feel badly that I was involved in failing to interpret a chest X ray and that in the heat of trying to respond to the cardiac arrest I did not have the clarity of mind to think of a possible pneumothorax. In all probability a more skilled trauma team might have recognized it. But, damnit, I am not going to compound my mistake by participating in a manipulation of the data so that it shows what we all know is not true."

"You are not going to compound your mistake? What are you going to do, Dr. Huntington, call in the media and commit professional suicide on the six-o'clock news?"

"Well, I—"

"Or are you hoping that you will be so admired for being honest that other job offers are going to come flowing in? Well, you can forget that. If you go out there and smear the name of this hospital, you'll still have me to deal with. You screw us and you won't be able to find a job in a tuberculosis ward in Africa. You understand me?"

Anthony straightened his tie. He walked to one of the steel cabinets, peered at his distorted reflection, and ran a comb through his hair. "I'll go through it again, and you people had better remember what I'm saying. The chopper crashed because the pilot had distorted his credentials on his résumé. The mayor was brought here in record time. Though he looked stable at the scene and even during the first few minutes he was in the emergency room, he had apparently suffered massive internal injuries. He was seen by a skilled emergency-room physician who quickly recognized the seriousness of his situation and who, within minutes, had notified a surgeon and had prepared the mayor for surgery. An equally skilled surgical team attended the mayor, but, despite their best efforts, the mayor succumbed to a major heart attack within minutes of arriving in the operating room. His heart simply couldn't tolerate the injury and the surgery."

"That sounds like a press release to me," Cummings said.

"If that's the way you want to look at it, it is. In any case, it is what I will say at the press conference I'm going to call for the morning and it would make life a lot easier for all of us if that were reflected in the postmortem examination report. Understood?" Anthony stared hard at every person in the room, not loosening the grip in his eyes until he had received an acquiescing nod from the pathologist, Harper, and Cummings. Then he turned his attention to the emergency-room physician.

"Huntington, is there anything in the pilot's medical condition that is likely to give us a problem?" Anthony questioned.

"No, he's fine. He should be out of here in a couple of days."

"Couple of days, nothing. I'm going to see to it that he's out of here by discharge time in the morning. In the meantime I am putting you in charge of seeing to it that the records clearly show that the mayor suffered massive internal injuries and that appropriate treatment was performed. Nothing that would even hint of anything to the contrary needs to be salvaged."

As Anthony spoke, Huntington slowly shook his head, refusing to meet the administrator's glance, choosing instead to stare past Anthony at the shrouded form of the mayor.

10

Julie, her elbows on her knees, her hands supporting her face, was watching Allan as he approached his apartment building.

"Uh-oh," he said, slowing his pace as he neared her. "Dinner."

"Dinner is right, Dr. Kirk. You were supposed to pick me up three hours ago. What the heck happened?"

Allan sat down next to her on the stoop and leaned back on the step behind them. "I'm sorry. I was at the lab and I just plain forgot. No excuses." He straightened and leaned over to kiss her. She kissed him back, then pulled away to look at him more carefully.

"The blood?"

"Yes, the blood. I've been going over and over that biker's death in my mind and I just couldn't come up with anything that would make it seem reasonable that the artificial blood killed him. I went in this morning at six and pulled the records on every animal we ever transfused with the artificial blood. I went over their autopsy reports line by line. I checked and rechecked lab values on the tests we ran while the animals were alive. I looked at microscopic sections of heart muscle tissues. Nothing. Normal. I looked at cross sections from pulmonary veins and lung sections from dozens of animals. No signs of anatomical compromise. I went over a hundred EKGs. Not the slightest hint that there were any problems with the electrical conduction system while the dogs had the artificial blood running through them. There was nothing there, Julie. Not one hint of anything that would indicate that the blood would affect heart function. The artificial blood didn't kill that kid, Julie. Coit Hill's half-assed emergency response system killed him."

Julie nodded. Then she asked suddenly, "By the way, if you were buried in that lab of yours all day, does that mean you didn't hear what happened to the mayor?"

"No, I heard."

"Can you believe it?"

"All I know is that the mayor is the least of my concerns at the moment."

Julie reached for his right hand and cupped it in her hands. He leaned closer to her. For five minutes they sat staring out at the nearly empty street.

"Even if I beat that artificial blood lawsuit, that is not the end of this nightmare."

"You'll get your department back, Allan. When things get back to an equilibrium neither Dorr nor the University will ask you to resign. They're just interested in punishing you."

"It's not that. Cummings has hit with another five malpractice lawsuits."

"Is he crazy?"

"He's not crazy. Anyway, he's just Anthony's hit man. They're out to destroy me, Julie. Completely. If Dorr hadn't already suspended me because I used the blood on the kid and because of my little speech before the Joint Committee for Emergency Services, these suits would have done the trick. The University lawyers have gone absolutely bananas over them."

"And you?"

"I was upset when they served me with the papers for the second suit. But when I got notice of the third, the fourth, and then the fifth suit, well, you know, it was like it wasn't real anymore. I figured if I don't beat the first one, the others won't matter anyway."

"Allan, why don't we go up to Napa Valley for a few days? Just take off and get away from San Francisco, from trauma, from Anthony. Let's just get out."

"I don't know. What if . . . ?"

"If what? If the University sends a delegation on its knees to beg you to come back?" She put her hand to the back of his neck and gently stroked beneath his hair. "Allan."

"I know. Forget I said it." He raised his arms high above his head and arched his back, stretching his muscles. He locked his fingers together and pushed his hands up even farther. He heard soft, dull cracks come from his knuckles, his neck, his shoulders, even his spine. "All right. What time should we leave in the morning?"

"The morning, nothing. We're leaving right now." Julie sprang to her feet, grabbed his hand, and pulled him up.

"Julie . . ."

"I don't want to hear about it. Go upstairs, throw some of your things into a bag, then let's go get my stuff and we're gone."

"What about your job?" Allan protested, more for show than effect.

"I'll call in and say I have to take care of a sick friend. And I won't be lying."

Forty-five minutes later, they were crossing the Oakland Bay Bridge. Julie turned in her seat and saluted the mini-Manhattan skyline along the city's waterfront. She kicked off her shoes, stretched to plant a wet, heavy kiss on Allan's cheek, and then sat back, tucking her legs under her. "We're gonna have one good time," she crowed. Allan laughed, despite himself.

Yountville, the small town Julie had suggested as their destination, was wrapped in the silence of the night. There were no people on the sidewalks, no cars driving through the streets. Every gas station was closed, as was every convenience store. After forty-five minutes of driving around, just as they were about to head farther north to the more touristy town of St.

Helena, Julie spied a small brick-and-fieldstone building. A small sign identified it as the Butterworth Inn.

Although light was shining through only one window, Allan pulled to the curb in front of the building. Julie jumped out, quietly opened the low iron gate, and walked up the stairs to the glass and wooden door. She turned the knob and gave the door a gentle push. It opened, and as she walked in she gestured to Allan to come up. When Allan joined her, a luggage bag in each hand, he felt as if he had stepped back in time. There was a gaslight ambiance to the small inn's reception area, a room that could have passed for the drawing room of a turn-of-the-century home. Only the small but conventional hotel front desk to their left and the morose, unshaven young man sitting behind it belied the impression that at any moment several women in bustles and high-necked dresses and men sporting generous mustaches and wearing spats, vests, and high tight collars would come in to have a tea.

"The Chardonnay room is available," the clerk told them in response to their inquiry for a room.

"The Chardonnay room?" Allan asked.

"Our rooms don't have numbers," the clerk answered with a touch of condescension. "We've named each one after a wine."

"Oh," was all Allan could manage in response as he picked up the key proffered him by the clerk.

"Your room is to the right of the stairs," the young man continued. "A complimentary breakfast is served at eight-thirty. The dining room is to the left on this floor, just below your room, in fact. Please be on time."

They climbed the narrow stairs and looked around. There were four rooms on the floor. Hanging from a nail on the door of three of the rooms were miniature pillows embroidered with the words "Quiet Please." The pillow on the fourth door read "Chardonnay Room." Allan tiptoed to one of the other doors and delicately turned over the pillow. "This," he whispered to Julie, "is the Cabernet room."

The "Chardonnay" was small and cozy. It too was furnished in the style of the late 1890s. There was a small antique end table. The high bed was covered with a generous quilt and at least half a dozen delicately embroidered pillows. An old-fashioned rag doll slumped comfortably on top of the heap. Curtains with delicately embroidered edges framed the one window. A white-and-light-blue color scheme dominated the room.

"A real pussy room," Allan snickered as he walked to the end table where he had noticed a crystal carafe of wine and two delicate glasses.

"Pig!" Julie said, throwing a pillow at him, which struck his shoulder.

Allan laughed. He pulled the stopper off the carafe and brought it to his nose. "Sherry, I think," he said as he carefully filled each glass halfway. He brought one over to Julie and sat down next to her on the bed. "To what?"

She kissed him lightly on the lips. "To the world that's just this room," she said and kissed him again.

They had not bothered to draw the blind and Julie, who was facing the window, was awakened by the bright sun shining through the voile curtains. Allan lay on his back, sound asleep, his head turned toward her, his face serene and relaxed. She reached out and with the index and middle finger of her right hand gently stroked his face. His light breathing continued to come in soft, rhythmic puffs. She ran her hand to his neck, caressed him there, moved on to the back of his shoulders. He shifted and, without waking up, moved onto his side so that he was facing Julie.

She propped herself up on her elbow. As she ran her hand lightly over his chest, she looked down. There was no sign that he was reacting to her. She moved her hand farther down, slowly moving it back and forth along the lower part of Allan's abdomen. Almost unnoticeably he moved his pelvis toward her. When she began to lightly stroke his thigh, he began to stir. As she watched him grow firmer and firmer she could feel an increasingly demanding pulsing in her groin. Abandoning subtlety, she reached for him. Almost in conjunction with her first firm upward stroke on him his eyes flew open. A puzzled look flitted across his face, as if the woman close to him were a stranger he had picked up the previous evening and whose name he could not now remember.

Quickly Allan broke into full consciousness and, with both

hands, pulled Julie's face toward his. She stroked faster and heatedly now as he squeezed her breasts, then ran his hand down her body. When he felt her urgent need, he pushed her on her back and mounted her. At first only the springs on the old bed creaked the steady cadence of love. But soon enough the bed's high brass frame began to beat against the wall behind it. The creaking and the drumming grew increasingly intense, increasingly quick, then stopped almost as abruptly as they had begun.

"Good morning," she said quietly as she caressed the back of Allan's head. "What time is it?" she added after Allan had responded with an indeterminate grunt.

He reached for his watch, which he had put on the floor next to his side of the bed. "We've got exactly seven minutes to get downstairs for breakfast, that's what time it is."

The dining room was barely larger than their room. Copper utensils and plates hung on the wood beams that were only partially embedded in the whitewashed walls. There were three heavy oak tables in the room and the Butterworth Inn's other guests were already seated around them. When Julie and Allan appeared in the doorway, the low hum of the conversation stopped.

"Oh, God," Julie said, squeezing Allan's hand.

Allan, who had seen two or three people bite their lips to keep from laughing, didn't have to ask Julie what her exclamation meant. "I wonder how many of those copper plates we shook off the wall," he said as they walked, trying to be as casual as possible, to the only table that had two unoccupied seats.

Julie flashed the other people the most innocent, carefree smile she could muster, "Well, what's for breakfast?" she asked lightly. It was a remark she regretted immediately when one of the other women at the table quickly rose and, shoulders shaking with barely concealed convulsions of laughter, headed for the door marked "Women" at the other side of the room.

After a hurried breakfast, they took time to wander through Yountville's streets. Stopping at a small wine-and-cheese shop, they bought an assortment of cheeses and an imported salami. At a bakery they found fresh bread. Before returning to the car, they made a quick visit to a supermarket to buy paper plates, plastic wineglasses, and an assortment of utensils, including a corkscrew for the bottle of wine they planned to pick up later for their picnic.

As they drove slowly away from Yountville, it didn't take them long to realize that this was the first time they had been able to be together under circumstances free of tension or pressure. As they covered back roads or stopped to sample the offerings of the smaller vintners (they had decided to avoid the larger wineries), they talked easily. Because of the fierce dedication with which he had thrown himself into trauma surgery, Allan had not had a serious and lasting relationship with a woman since medical school and he found himself almost babbling in his desire to talk to Julie about anything that came into his mind. He was surprised at his own eagerness to communicate, to talk about everything and anything, ranging from the oppressive and complex relationship he had with his father to the most trivial of events in his life. He found himself trying hard to remember events that he could toss out for Julie's consideration.

Allan's willingness to open his life to her made Julie happy. Although they were lovers, she still harbored strong doubts about the depth of Allan's commitment to her and had been steeling herself for the possibility that if Allan's troubles waned, he would fade from her life and immerse himself again in his much-beloved trauma team at the University. Now that he was opening up to her, the relationship was being reinforced by ties that, at least in her mind, insured that they would be more than casual lovers.

At the same time, Julie felt that now she too could open herself to him. She had kept herself physically, intellectually, and emotionally isolated since her fiancé's death. Once she had managed to make love with Allan, she had been glad that with his help she had broken out of her physical isolation. And now, as they drove through the countryside, in response to his offerings, she too offered glimpses of her inner life. She was trusting a relationship for the first time in three years.

Their conversation had turned to a lighter vein when they stumbled, accidentally, on the Lower Creek Winery—a winery not identified on their small guide map of all of the Napa Valley wineries. It was located on what Allan described as a "back back road," one they had turned into by mistake.

The main building, which seemed to be a medium-sized barn, stood about one hundred feet off the highway and was reached by another, narrower, gravel-topped road. They walked through a corrugated-iron door into a large, dimly lit hall. To their left and straight ahead stood row upon row of massive oak barrels. To their right was a counter. Julie smiled. "I love that sweet smell of the wine and the smell of the oak that hits you in these small places," she whispered. "Smell!"

A short man, about sixty, was standing behind the counter, one hand flat against the wood, the other wrapped about an open bottle of wine.

"Zo?" he asked in a slight German accent.

The tall, thin, slightly stooped man on the customer side of the counter nodded vigorously. His hollow cheeks were covered by gray stubble. His eyes said that he had been sampling wine here since the early hours of the day. "It is good, I have told you that before," the stooped man said. "It is not surprising, eh? They are my grapes, eh? Do I sell you grapes that would not make a good wine?" He too spoke with a foreign intonation.

Absentmindedly, the owner turned to Julie and Allan, placing two glasses before them. Unlike the hosts at other wineries who had poured them only half-inch samples of the wines they wanted to try, the Lower Creek man gave them almost a quarter of a glass each. Allan looked at a blackboard bearing the names of the various wines made here and reasoned that if they sampled them all at the owner's generous dispensations, they would probably have to plan on sleeping the afternoon away on the floor between the barrels.

The owner watched them sip. "Good, yes?" He motioned with the bottle toward the other man. "This refugee from Alsace-Lorraine thinks I make good wines because he sells me grapes. But it is what you do with the grapes that is the most important." He motioned with the bottle again, this time toward the barrels around him. He leaned forward, placing the cork back in the bottle. "Everybody wants to make a lot of wine fast and cheap.

They put it in big aluminum casks. Idiots. Ach!" he said, punching the cork vehemently into place. "That was my Gewurtztraminer. Want to try the Chardonnay?"

Near an aging walnut tree, they spread out Allan's well-worn but still serviceable army blanket, then neatly arranged their foods and utensils on it. Allan opened the wine and poured generous measures into the plastic wineglasses. That done, they sat down and, in almost complete silence, polished off the provisions they had brought along.

Allan poured himself another glass of wine, then tried to make himself comfortable against the gnarled trunk of the tree that shaded their picnic. Julie leaned her head on his leg and stretched out. With exaggerated ceremony she popped grapes into her mouth. Allan cut an apple into small sections and dipped each slice into his wine before taking a bite from it. When he had eaten the last bit of his apple, he raided Julie's grape cluster for a handful of individual grapes. The wine, the sun, Julie's nearness warmed him. He felt content.

"Well," he said with a gigantic sigh. "What do you think I ought to do?"

"I dunno. How about going to Africa and taking up where Doc Schweitzer left off?"

"I'm serious, Julie," he said quietly. "We've avoided talking about this for—"

"Then why spoil the day?"

"Not spoiling it. But, maybe it's the wine, I feel I can talk about it objectively now, like it's a thing that is removed from me."

"You're welcome to think that. But I wouldn't go around making decisions about the rest of my life in some cow pasture, after half a day of wine tasting."

"I'm serious."

"Okay." She reached up to stroke his cheek. "I don't know what there is to talk about. This will blow over. It may take six months, a year, but it'll pass. Then you'll go on working at the University or do whatever it is you had planned on doing before your big mouth got you in trouble."

"I wish it were that pat. Trouble is, I'm scared it won't blow over. And if it doesn't, I just don't have a lot of options left. I know you think it's all temporary, but, whenever I think of losing the trauma department I want to cry. And I mean that: I've come damned close to just breaking down and bawling."

She said nothing.

"And what options have I got if it doesn't blow over?"

"Come on, Allan. You could go into private practice."

"Private practice? Become a general surgeon and spend the rest of my life dealing with hernias, hemorrhoids, and hysterectomies? I can just see myself joining the county medical association and going on their 'Moonlight Magic Bay Cruises' or to their little dances so I can suck up to internists in the hope that they might refer cases to me."

"It's not that bad."

"No, it's worse. I could spare myself that and go to work for some health-maintenance organization. What a prospect that is. A medical civil servant, working nine to five, making decisions based not on medicine but on rules, regulations, and guidelines, trying to decide whether surgery is really recommended for my patient or whether the operation would just be a needless expense that would lower profits for the group and therefore cut into my profit sharing."

"All right, if any sort of practice except trauma disgusts you so much, then fend your mences. God, the wine has gotten me too. I mean, mend your fences. Take the advice Dorr gave you. Go into a low profile the hunchback of Notre Dame would envy. Don't do interviews, don't do death studies. Bury yourself in that lab of yours with all those dogs you're torturing in the name of humanity and don't come out until Dorr sends for you and lets you out of irons."

They lapsed into silence again. Allan stared into the ruby-colored liquid left in his glass, moved his wrist, causing the wine to swirl around its sides. Julie munched on her grapes.

"You've got another option."

"Which is?"

"Fight back."

"And what will that get me except guarantee me the University's undying enmity?"

"Oh, I'm not so sure that it is very easy to do that. You know, essentially you've got a bunch of spineless people up there. It's ridiculous. Those people have a responsibility to the community and beyond that to the people whose taxes allow them to crap around in a relatively carefree fashion. When you recognize a major and important problem in the community and suggest a change, they run for cover the first time Anthony makes a little noise. So maybe the thing to do is to fight back, to stand up for your rights, to stand up for the rights of all those trauma patients of yours. I bet if you make a little more noise than Anthony, if you take him on, they'll cave in to you. You have to decide to what lengths you want to go and whether you can take more of the crap Anthony might dish up. But if you decide to do it, I bet you can whip him."

"Holy cow, Julie. Have you considered becoming a football coach?"

She scrambled to her feet, then knelt to face him. "I'm serious, Allan."

He reached out and drew her to him. "I know. It's just that it sounds so impossible."

Julie freed herself from his embrace. "That was just one possibility. I'll help you whatever you decide to do, even if it is to just go on being your own unpredictable, erratic self."

Two days later they arrived back in San Francisco. It was near midnight.

"What are you going to do tomorrow, then?" Julie asked as Allan slowed the car and pulled to the curb in front of her apartment.

"Go back to the lab. Go over some more of the artificial blood stuff."

"I thought you had convinced yourself that it had nothing to do with the biker's death."

"I am convinced. But it's not just a question of convincing myself. I'm going to have to convince a jury and that'll be tougher."

Julie kissed him lightly on the lips, then pulled back slightly. "Want to spend the night?"

Allan put his hand on the back of her head, drew her back toward him, and kissed her. "No, not tonight. I want to go over some data I have at home before I go to the lab in the morning. I was going to do that the night we left for Napa."

Julie kissed him, then reached into the backseat for her bag. "Okay," she said mockingly, "but I think it's awfully early in the relationship for me to start being a work widow." She opened the door, put one leg out, then looked back at him. "Call me tomorrow?"

"Plan on dinner. Call me at the lab to remind me in case I get wrapped up again."

Fifteen minutes later, Allan was at home. He unpacked only his toilet kit, gave his teeth a quick brushing, and headed for his desk and the reams of computer sheets on it.

At 7:30 the next morning, Allan walked into the building that housed his laboratory, a red brick structure set in a grove of towering eucalyptus trees. The old building was the original site of the University hospital but had been abandoned as the importance and reputation of the medical center spread. Because it was no longer the main part of the center's life and because it was so early in the morning, the halls were deserted. He relished the thought of having an hour or two for himself before the kibitzers—or at least those who had ignored the rumblings about him—started stopping by to exchange gossip or seek another opinion on their personal or research problems. But as he slowly walked toward his laboratory, he heard an uncharacteristic amount of noise—hammering, sawing—coming from that part of the floor where his lab was located. He quickened his step and turned a corner.

He stopped, stunned by the scene in front of him. His first thought was that he had stumbled upon a burglary team intent on stealing whatever possible from his lab. Microscopes, his centrifuge machine, the highly sensitive blood analysis machine, the gas spectograph were lined up in a neat row along one wall leading away from the laboratory door. Crates, boxes, and files were lined up along the left wall. The cages in which he had kept his experimental dogs were stacked against the wall opposite his door. The cages were empty.

Frightened, he broke into a trot. When he reached the laboratory, he saw that the "burglars" were men from the hospital's building-services department. He pushed a workman aside and almost fell into the laboratory. Everything had been changed. Shelves were going up where the dog cages had been. A substantial part of the lab had simply been gutted and a new room divider was being put in place.

He grabbed a man trying to walk by him. "What gives, man?"

The worker freed himself. "I sure as shit don't know, buddy. Just doing what I was told to do."

Crazed, Allan looked around, trying to latch onto someone who had some authority, who could tell him why his lab was being taken apart.

The man he had stopped, somehow deciding that maybe Allan had some right to know what the crew was doing, pointed at a tall, heavyset man who was standing in the middle of the erstwhile lab, chewing on a toothpick and drinking coffee from a Styrofoam cup. "That's the foreman over there, fella. Ask him."

In three steps Allan stood in front of the man. "I'm Dr. Kirk. This is my lab. May I ask what is going on here?"

Without bothering to speak, the foreman stuck out his right index finger and, flicking his wrist back and forth, pointed behind Allan. He turned around to see Jack White, the hospital administrator, framed in the doorway.

Allan kicked aside a box of nails and a toolbox that were in his way and marched to the door. "Jack, what is going on here?" he keened. "What are they doing to my lab?"

White stepped backward out of the door. "Let's go into your office and have a little talk." Allan didn't know whether to be angry at White's patronizing tone or to be relieved that his office was still in one piece. In silence they walked the fifty steps to the room he had been given to do his paperwork and keep his books and records. White sat down in one of the office's spartan metal folding chairs. Allan chose a chair across from him.

"Well?"

"Look, I don't know how to tell you any other way, so I'm just going to tell you straight out." He paused for a moment, looked down at the floor, then brought his eyes up to meet Allan's. "Your application for the renewal of your NIH grant has been turned down."

Allan stared at him as if White had said nothing, as if he were still waiting for the administrator's explanation.

"It's been turned down? That's impossible. Why would NIH turn down a proposal for a study they've been funding for five years just when it's about to come to fruition? What are you talking about?" Allan stopped, then flared. "White, if this is your—"

The administrator held up both hands, palms facing Allan. "Whoa, before you go off half-cocked in the wrong direction. I know we've had our differences, but I had nothing to do with this. Nothing."

"Then who else? I mean, my God, come to think of it, the grant wasn't going to be up for consideration for another six weeks, at the minimum. And besides, it was an automatic conclusion that at this point we would go on to clinical trials. Everybody's been saying that we have the best artificial blood product, that the Chicago group is six to nine months behind us. I mean, there's no way we could lose. The only way NIH would pull back is if they heard from this institution that people had grave doubts about what we were doing."

"Don't be naïve, Allan."

"Naïve? Naïve about what?"

"You mean you really don't know? Forty-eight hours after the lawsuit was filed by the people whose kid you had given the artificial blood to at Coit Hill, there were inspectors nosing around here. They talked to Dorr for hours, they interviewed half a dozen people. Almost everyone on the trauma teams."

"No one told me." Allan was flabbergasted. "So?" he finally added.

"They were Bumqua staffers."

Allan shook his head. "Wait. Wait a minute. What does Bumqua have to do with this? The Board of Medical Quality

Assurance is a California agency. Their big thing is to go after a few poor alcohol- or drug-addicted docs each year."

"Maybe they already got their cocaine-snorter quota for the year. I don't know. But I do know they're after you."

"Me?"

"You."

"Because of the lawsuits?"

"Not the other ones that have been filed. Because of the one actually involving your artificial blood. That's a lawsuit that alleges that you experimented on a live patient. Even assuming that he or his family could have given you valid consent to use a procedure that hasn't been approved for human experimentation, you didn't have that consent. There's a lot of sensitivity about that sort of thing."

Allan felt a heavy curtain of depression descend, and covered his face with his hands. "I still haven't gotten my answer about NIH, but never mind that for now. How did all this get to Bumqua's attention?"

"I would imagine they read the papers like everybody else." White paused for a moment, looked down at his highly shined shoes. Holding the heels together, he moved the shoes back and forth, back and forth like hedge clippers. "And if by chance they missed the story that morning, I'm sure that someone was more than glad to tip them off."

"Anthony!"

"You could never prove it. But . . ."

"That son of a bitch. That mother-fucking—"

"Come on, Allan, what did you expect? You think you were in the middle of some nice, tidy academic debate after which you and the others would go have a few friendly beers together? Come on, man. You were throwing stones at a heavyweight. Just what did you think would happen? I take it back. Knowing you, you never gave the consequences a moment's thought. They've gone for your jugular, Allan. You're going to learn the hard way."

"Okay. All right. Never mind the triumphant speech."

"Believe it or not, I'm not gloating. I don't much like you, but I wouldn't wish this on you."

Allan ignored the remark. "And NIH?"

"I don't know. Maybe when the Bumqua people found out you had an NIH grant they felt compelled to call Bethesda. Maybe Anthony tipped off the Feds too. In any case, it was a smart move. The Feds don't like to get involved in the middle of a sticky issue like this, especially not now that Congress is arguing over next year's budget and the Right-to-Lifers are going over everything with a magnifying glass to make sure that the government isn't killing babies or comatose patients. Anyway, when we received a phone call and then a telegram to inform us that funding for your project was suspended, Dorr wanted to reach you, but couldn't."

"I went up to Napa for a few days," Allan said. I was lying in pastures, trying to make believe I had a life left, he added silently to himself.

White pushed himself off the chair and placed it against the wall. "Look, I know it all looks hopeless now, but maybe you can ride this out. The worst that could happen is that you have to pick up a research project at another university and . . ."

Allan motioned him to stop. "If you don't mind, I'd better start gathering up some of the things I need before those guys ruin them." He started to get up from his chair, but found he couldn't. His legs, his body felt unbearably heavy. Worse, he felt paralyzed. Without trying to hide the state he was in, he looked up at White. "On second thought, just ask them to leave my stuff in the hall. I'll get it later."

White looked at him, unqualified sorrow in his eyes. He turned and, closing the door, quietly left.

Allan sat listening to the sounds of the building coming alive. Through the frosted window in the door he saw the hallway, which on his arrival had been dimly lit by auxiliary lights, burst into the white glare of fluorescent lighting. He watched shadows pass back and forth, some hurrying, others just loping along. On occasion two people stopped in front of his office and he watched, with detached curiosity, as they talked. Though he could hear sounds, he couldn't make out words. And even if he could have, he would not have listened. There came a time in the day when the hall was full of passing shadows, sometimes lone ones, sometimes in twosomes, sometimes in small groups, all headed in the same direction. A bit later, the shadows came back, this time heading in the opposite direction, at a slower, more leisurely pace. The lunch hour was over.

Once or twice in the afternoon, a shadow came to his door. The doorknob would turn one way, then the other. There would be a small, hesitant knock on the glass. Then the shadow would leave. Twice the phone rang. Once the caller waited for a full minute before deciding that there would be no answer. The second time, the phone rang only half a dozen times before the call was disconnected. When Allan was sure that there were no more shadows in the hall and when he saw the lights in the hallway dim in allegiance to the University's energy-saving program, he got up and walked out.

11

He was sleeping on his stomach, one arm and one leg hanging over the edge of the bed, when the ringing of the telephone, sounding distant and muffled, summoned him back to consciousness. He opened his eyes and looked down at the instrument sitting on the floor next to the bed. Making no attempt to move, he simply watched the telephone as it rang again and again. When it finally stopped, he slowly pushed himself off the bed, kicked aside an empty can of beer, and stumbled to the bathroom.

He was washing his face when the telephone began clamoring again. Angry, he slammed down his washcloth, stalked back into the bedroom, and snatched the telephone off its cradle.

"Yes," he yelled into the mouthpiece. "What is it?"

There was a silence at the other side. "One moment, please, Dr. Kirk," a woman said, her voice very discernibly tight as if she were trying hard to remain civil, "Dr. Dorr wishes to talk to you."

He heard the click of the hold button, then the onslaught of the local radio show given to "easy listening" music, entertainment the hospital thoughtfully patched in for callers asked to wait. Allan was moving the phone away from his ear, preparing to hang up, when Dorr came on the line.

"Allan, where in heaven's name have you been?"

"Nowhere in particular." Allan could find neither the energy nor the will to say more.

Dorr's voice was apologetic. "I'm sorry you had to find out about the lab the way you did. We tried to locate you when we first heard about NIH."

"So White said yesterday." Allan felt a sudden surge of anger and resentment. "How convenient that I was out of town when all this came down."

The implication was not lost on Dorr. "There was little you could have done if you had been here," Dorr said, choosing not to rise to the bait. "The Bumqua people were not ready to talk to you, they said they would be in touch with you in due time, and the NIH move was preemptory. They did not even seek our views before they took their action. Your presence might have softened the blow for you, but it would have done nothing to change the course of things."

Allan grunted.

"Retreating into a shell will accomplish nothing. You're in serious trouble, there is no denying that. But if you just, well, I don't know exactly what you are doing, but if you don't make at least a minimal attempt to participate in a resolution, then there is no chance at all that you'll salvage anything."

Allan, who had been standing, lowered himself slowly to his unkempt bed. "And where do you suggest I start, Phil? By calling Bethesda and begging? By going before the University board and begging? By—"

Dorr's voice was impatient now. "You can start by doing away with the self-pity! After all, you're not an innocent victim in this. There isn't a thing that's happening to you that isn't your own doing!"

Responding to the edge in Dorr's voice, Allan was for the moment goaded out of his gloom. "That might be true. Okay, it is true. But would you have let that kid die knowing that you had something in the trunk of your car that had an outside chance of saving him?"

"Allan . . ." Weariness now crept into Dorr's voice.

"Yes, maybe you would have. I know. Protocol. The

scientific method. The proper way of doing things. And what about those E.R. deaths? If you'd been privy to them, would you have kept quiet?" Sarcasm was winding into his voice. "Yes, come to think of it, I bet you would have. You sure as hell don't get to be chairman of the department of surgery at that place by taking chances and talking out of turn."

"Allan, that's enough!" Dorr paused for a moment to collect himself. "In any case, I called to let you know that we are going to try to come to some sort of understanding with the family of the boy who died after receiving your experimental artificial blood. There is going to be a preliminary meeting tomorrow in the main conference room at the hospital."

"An understanding? What are you talking about?"

"What I'm talking about is that no one wants to see this drag on for years. It is in no one's best interests."

"What you're saying is that you're looking for a settlement."

"No one's talking—"

"I mean that's what you want, isn't it? To get out from under. Right now. Jesus Christ almighty, you people don't even have the decency to wait—"

"Allan!" Dorr stopped again. "You somehow have to get it through that steel head of yours that this does not concern you alone. Whatever the great humanitarian feelings that led you to give that boy the artificial blood, you could be deemed an agent of the University and therefore you endangered the University."

"Oh, fuck the—"

"I've stuck by you through a lot. I have a lot invested in you, not just as a teacher who has had a soft spot for a brilliant but difficult child, but as a friend. Don't test it further, Allan. It's not just the artificial blood, either, for that matter. Now we've learned that Anthony has gone to the Board of Supervisors and underbid our contract for indigent care by a good half a million dollars. I don't know how he's going to do it, or what kind of care those people are going to get at Coit Hill Memorial. But I'll tell you one thing, if the Board of Supervisors accept his bid, we are in deep trouble. It will decimate our training program. And I'm not going to spare you that, either. That rests entirely on your shoulders as well. I am convinced that he bid for that contract for no other reason than the fact that you work for us."

Allan slowly slumped into a sitting position on the bed. "What do you want me to do, Phil? You want me to come to the front steps of the hospital, put the sword to my belly, and fall on it? Will that make things easier for all of you? Fine, I'll do that, Phil."

"Don't be a fool. But it might be a start to show up tomorrow, to at least start showing some concern, some . . ."

"Humility?"

"Call it what you want. I don't know what we can salvage out of all this for us, or for you, but an appearance would be a start." And with that, Dorr hung up.

For a moment Allan considered crawling back into bed, but he was tired of staying in bed and shuffled back to the bathroom instead to finish washing. He had no sooner reached the shower stall than the phone rang again. He turned and stared at it as if hoping that his very glare could snap the connection and spare him further contact with the outside world. But though he was determined to stand his ground, apparently so was the caller. Defeated, he walked back and answered. It was Julie.

"Allan, my gosh, I've been calling since noon yesterday. What is going on?"

He fought for control. The same question from anyone else would have been greeted by a hostile answer. The way she asked it, the frightened concern in her voice as if she already suspected the worst, rekindled in him the feeling that he had fallen into a hopeless abyss.

"Allan? Baby, what is it?"

"They've closed my lab." It came in a whisper, but she had heard. A sharp pain thrust through her stomach. "Someone called NIH, tipped them off. Someone called the Board of Medical Quality Assurance. They're looking into my license."

Julie felt the room spin around her. She leaned forward in her chair and leaned her elbow on her paper-cluttered desk. She propped her head on her hand. "I'll finish up here and come over."

"No!" He was surprised himself by the harshness in the word. "I'm sorry, I didn't mean to shout. I just want to be by myself, not think about anything, not make any plans. I'm tired, Julie. I'm awfully tired."

Julie closed her eyes and tried hard to choose the right words. "Let's have some coffee somewhere, let's talk."

"There's not much to talk about right now, Julie. I—"

"Allan, don't pull back from me. I can help you on this, sweetheart. Don't try to fight it out yourself."

"Julie, just for now, for today." Despite his self-preoccupation he could feel her foreboding. "Too much has been going on and I have to sort it out. By myself."

"Will you call?"

The plea brought him further out of himself. "I'm not splitting, Julie." He thought for a moment. "There's some kind of a meeting at the University tomorrow morning about the lawsuit. I'll call you afterward."

"Okay," she said, though she did not sound at all convinced.

The city editor of the *Telegraph*, Carroll Vanowen, sauntered over to Younger's desk and drew up a chair. He turned it around and straddled it, placing his arms on its back. He flashed Younger an ingratiating smile, replete with perfectly lined and shiny teeth. "How'ya doing?" he asked lightly.

"Just fine," Younger answered, consciously trying to imitate Vanowen's tone. He could hardly wait to hear what press conference, called by some minor pharmaceutical house to announce the twentieth cure for herpes, Vanowen would ask him to cover now.

But Vanowen surprised him. "What do you know about our good mayor's death?"

Younger, who had been slouching, sat up. "Just what I read in the papers."

"You haven't had any reason to think we should have looked harder at the circumstances of his death?"

Younger, who had acted as the lead reporter on the story, was tempted to be insulted, but decided against it. "No, nothing. They did an autopsy immediately after he died at the hospital and the pathologist's report said he died as a result of a myocardial infarction, complicated by extensive internal injuries."

"Why wasn't there an official postmortem? Isn't the county Medical Examiner required to do one in every case like this?"

"What the hell is all this about? There were a dozen stories about all of this after the accident."

"Just hold on. Why wasn't an official post done?"

"By law, the coroner is supposed to do a post in every case where the underlying cause of death needs to be clarified. But by and large they do those when a hospital pathologist hasn't done a postmortem, which is most of the time because the hospital has no inherent interest in doing them in most cases. But in the mayor's case, the hospital did, because obviously they had to have some answers to explain his death. So the M.E.'s office took their word for it. The guy who did it at Coit Hill acted as a deputy coroner and is board certified. He's got a pretty good rep around town, so—"

"What about the coroner's inquest? One of your stories mentioned that possibility."

"Never came to that. The weight of all the investigations were on the crash itself and since those proved that it was just an accident and that the pilot was at fault, no one saw any reason to bother with a death caused by a plunging helicopter."

Vanowen wheeled his chair closer to Younger. "What do you think? You're the trauma expert around here."

"You still haven't—"

"Stay with me a minute more. What do you think?"

"I don't know. The pilot who also went to Coit Hill Memorial survived, so that's an argument for the fact that they received proper care there. On the other hand, the talk is that Coit Hill Memorial can't get its docs to really support its so-called trauma center, so it could be that other factors contributed to the mayor's death."

"Like?"

"Like the usual. That they couldn't get anyone in to operate on the sucker. Or they got someone who didn't know what to do."

"Can you prove any of that?"

"It would be tough. You'd have to be able to see the medical records from start to finish and have them evaluated by someone who would look at all the line-by-line entries and tell you what care he got or didn't get and why or why not."

"Can you try to get them?"

"I guess. But why? Did we get another hot, but anonymous, conspiracy-tip call on the city desk?"

"No. But I was at a cocktail party last night. I only knew a couple of people, so, you know how these things go, I wandered from group to group. I got into one group because there were a couple of real dolls. I talked to them, but at the same time was listening to a couple of guys there yacking about what a downer the E.R. department at Coit Hill Memorial is these days and how this guy Huntington is barely fit to live with since the mayor's death there."

"And you think that bears checking out?"

Vanowen cocked an eyebrow.

Younger picked up a pencil and drummed its eraser against his desk. "Well, Pulitzers have been built on thinner leads. I'll take a whack at it."

His first call was to the University's public-information office. The public relations woman was cheery and helpful while giving him the details she had been authorized to release on the condition of Supervisor Page, namely, that despite his widespread injuries he was doing well.

"Who treated him when he first came in?" Younger asked. "Was it Dr. Kirk?"

There was, to the reporter's practiced ear, a significant pause at the other end. "As you know, Sam, the hospital's trauma service is based on a system of teams. No particular doctor is assigned to any particular case."

"Yeah. But you haven't answered my question. Did Kirk work on the supervisor?"

She was all business now. "I'm sorry, but I don't have that information at my disposal."

"You're bullshitting me, Jenny, but thanks anyway." Younger hung up.

He picked through one of the three telephone number indexes he kept on his desk until he found Allan's card. There was no answer at his home. There was no answer at his lab. He called the emergency room. He was told they did not know his whereabouts. He replaced the receiver. He stood, buttoned up his vest, and, grabbing his tape recorder and two tapes, left the newsroom.

Allan's office was locked. Dorr would not talk to him, even off the record. Younger prowled about the University's emergency room until he found a nurse on a coffee break in the lounge. "You're not going to find Dr. Kirk around here," she told him. "Rumor is he got canned. Closed his lab too."

For a moment Younger considered going back to the paper just to write the story of Allan's firing. But he decided it would hold until he dug up more information, and took a cab to Coit Hill Memorial. He hung around the emergency room, chatted with some nurses and the emergency doctor on call, telling them that he was gathering material for a feature on trauma care. He learned nothing, even when he casually mentioned the mayor's stay in the E.R. None of the people he talked to had been on duty that day. But twenty minutes after he had arrived, one of Coit Hill Memorial's public relations people arrived on the scene to see if she "could be of help." When he asked to talk to Anthony she told him the administrator was in a long series of meetings and could not be disturbed. When he mentioned he wanted to talk to Huntington, she told him that the doctor was busy organizing a major conference on trauma and had asked not to be made available for interviews for at least several weeks. Then, smiling all the way, she escorted him out the door.

Younger stood outside the hospital's front door, weighing his options and deciding that he really didn't have many. Maybe, he thought, he should just go back to the paper and tell Vanowen to keep his hunches to himself. But then he looked at his watch and decided that he had time to take a few more stabs at trying to find if there were something to the young city editor's suspicions.

The black woman at the reception counter at the medical examiner's office greeted him like an old friend. "How you doing, Sam Younger? Another hot story?"

"No story yet, kid. Just another editor's bright idea."

Casually, he made for the revolving file on the desk to her left. It had multiple aluminum flaps, each one containing a long vertical row of thin individual slips of paper. Each slip contained the name of a man, woman, or child who had been the subject of an autopsy in the last year. The slip also listed a file number, one in which the autopsy results could be found. The guide was there as a service to police officers, criminal law lawyers, and other attorneys representing families of people who had died and who had need for an autopsy report.

Younger silently cursed himself for being at the morgue, for taking up time that would be better spent working on other stories. Why would anything be in there about the mayor, he asked himself. He had already given Vanowen good reasons why the mayor would not have been the subject of an autopsy here. The reasons were no less valid now. There would be no listing of the mayor's name. No file number. Nothing.

The mayor's name, last name first, was neatly typed on a slip, filed amid the usual contingent of "Does, John" and "Does, Jane" who had died and had been hauled to the medical examiner's office on the same day as the accident.

Younger made out the call slip required to retrieve the file and walked over to the woman behind the desk. Somehow, the woman had never questioned his right to see files when he asked for them. But because of the case involved he was careful to act no differently than he did on any of his other visits here. "You mind digging this one out for me? I'm sort of on a deadline."

She regarded him with mock exasperation. "Has there ever been a time when you were in here and *not* on a deadline?"

She was back within a few minutes. "Sorry, Sam, the file is out."

Younger cursed under his breath. "Who has it?"

She looked at a large yellow card in her hand. Each side of the card had about a dozen horizontal lines on it and three vertical sections. The clerk looked at the last line. "Julie McDonough."

"Who's she?"

"The statistician here."

Younger scratched the back of his head. "She in?"

"She hasn't been around all day. And, no, I'm not going to tell you her home phone number."

He took a taxi back to the paper and went to the newspaper's library. He stepped up to a video display terminal on one of the three desks reserved for reporters who needed to do research in the newspaper's files and called up the name index to the library's holdings. When he saw Julie's name listed, he punched the keys that would bring the story in which she had been mentioned to the screen. It was a five-paragraph story detailing an accident a few years earlier on a Twin Peaks street. She was listed as a survivor. No address was given. Oh, for the good old days, Younger said to himself, when leaving someone's address out of a story, even a five-paragraph story, was grounds for dismissal.

The telephone book was no help. There were fifteen McDonough's listed and, judging from the fact that five of the listings carried only the initial J. and a phone number without a corresponding street address, he surmised that the five were women.

He looked at his watch. Rather than make five probably useless calls to find the right J. McDonough, he dialed the motor-vehicle license department in Sacramento and asked for a clerk with whom he had dealt before.

"Who you lookin' for this time?" the man asked after they had exchanged pleasantries.

"I'm looking for McDonough, Julie."

"Another chick that wouldn't give you her phone number in a bar, huh? Hold on."

Younger held on.

"McDonough, Julie," the voice at the other end announced after a few minutes. "Nine-three-four–seven-seven-five-nine. Address: six twenty-one Polk."

"Thanks, George. You're a prince."

"Never mind the prince crap. Just remember me when there's an extra ticket for a Forty-niners game this fall," George retorted.

"You just call and name the date and I'll have two for you," Younger answered happily.

The moment she opened the door he recognized her as the woman who had been with Allan at the stormy meeting of the Joint Committee for Emergency Services. This woman, he said to himself, has been doing some crying.

"I'm Sam Younger. I'm with the *Telegraph*," he said as he pulled out his press card.

Julie looked at it. "So?"

"I'm trying to find Dr. Kirk. Any idea where he is?"

"I haven't talked to him since earlier in the day." Julie was wary. "If you'll excuse me . . ." She began to close the door.

Younger put his hand on the door. "Ms. McDonough, just a couple of minutes. It really is important."

She hesitated, then pulled the door open. "All right, come in, but just for a few minutes."

Younger followed her in to the kitchen where she had been having a cup of coffee. He saw an open folder on the kitchen table. The markings identified it as a file from the medical examiner's office. She offered him coffee, brought it over and sat down.

He decided to plunge in. "Ms. McDonough, was Dr. Kirk fired from the University?"

The look of anger that flashed across her face immediately made him regret the question. Without giving Julie a chance to answer, he added, "I might be able to help." If Julie and Allan were more than just casual acquaintances and if the nurse at the University had been right about Allan's dismissal, then the distress he saw in Julie was probably rooted in her concern for his well-being. He would not get any information out of her, he reasoned, unless he could make some gesture that would show he could be of value to her and Allan.

"Sure you'll help," Julie said. "Out of the kindness of your heart."

"Not entirely. I think the story is important, that people should know what is going on in the medical community. But if I can help Kirk in the process of putting the story together, so much the better."

Julie said nothing. Younger decided to take her silence as acceptance of his offer and a plan began to form in his mind.

Younger pointed at the medical examiner's file on the table. "The mayor's records?"

"Yes," Julie answered softly.

"You brought them home to see if there was something there that would help?"

"I was trying to think of something. I know how Allan feels about Coit Hill Memorial. I thought there'd be something in there that would help."

"And?"

She pushed the folder at him. "This was not even supposed to be at the office because we didn't post him. But I guess someone at the hospital just decided to follow routine and sent over what records were available. They send stuff over when they don't have to and don't send it when it is important."

Younger opened it. Inside was a single sheet of paper, a summary of the pathologist's report saying that the mayor had suffered several rib fractures, severe lacerations of the liver, and coronary occlusive disease with evidence of acute myocardial ischemia and infarction. The injuries were exactly as described by hospital spokesmen to the press.

"That's it?" he asked. "No. E.R. charts? No O.R. records?"

"Nothing."

"Well, let's see then what I can do." He reached into the left inside pocket of his jacket and pulled out a thick personal phone book. "Last year I wrote a series of stories about efforts to water down the certification processes for out-of-state nurses who want to come to California," he explained to Julie as he thumbed through the book. "The woman who was president of the California Professional Nurses Society was able to use the articles to lobby against the efforts in the legislature. Maybe she knows somebody on the inside at Coit Hill who can shed some light on all this."

He dialed a number and began to talk into the phone. After a few minutes, he made notes on his pad, thanked the person he was speaking to and hung up.

"I reached the Nurses Society president. She says she'll check around, but she's already pretty sure she knows a nurse who works the emergency room at Coit. She'll call her and try to set up an interview with her for me."

Julie looked at him with suspicion. "Is that for real?"

"Absolutely. She may come up empty-handed, but she'll try. The media doesn't have a terrific reputation with the public at large. But there are people who learn to trust us . . . and to help us because we've helped them. She might lead us to some useful information." He stopped to let his words sink in. "Now, what can you tell me about what has been happening to Dr. Kirk?"

Julie poured more coffee for them. Then, starting with the biker's death at Coit Hill, began to tell him what had happened to Allan.

Allan had slept fitfully, waking every hour or so to determine what time it was. Finally, at six, he dragged himself out of bed, took a shower, and shaved. As he slapped on after-shave and looked at himself in the mirror, he realized that the struggle over the last few weeks—and the confrontation with the dismantling of his lab in particular—had taken a heavy toll. His eyes were sunk even deeper in his face and there were even darker shadows underneath them. His normally thin face looked more drawn than usual. If he were in bed in an oncology ward, he thought, any reasonable passerby would assume that he was terminal. He was not surprised when he stepped on the scale he kept below the sink and found that he had lost some ten pounds since he had last weighed himself at the beginning of the month.

Out of the bottom drawer of his dresser he drew a white shirt, inspected it to make sure that the collar was not excessively frayed and that it had all its buttons, then put it on. He slipped into a pair of pressed chino slacks he kept in the closet for dress-up emergencies, quickly knotted a tie, and walked out the door. He was halfway down the stairs when he realized he had forgotten his coat.

He was at the University by 8:30 and, rather than confront the staff parking lot, he pulled into the lot for visitors. When he had shut off the ignition, he briefly considered staying in his car until a few minutes before nine, but dismissed the idea. Coming in so close to the starting time would put him in the position of walking into a room full of people who, to varying degrees, considered him the villain in the piece, the source of their problems. He decided he wanted to be there when the others arrived, as though he were just another participant interested in an equitable agreement. Besides, he reasoned, the morning meetings were always accompanied by juice, hot coffee, and pastry. And since he had not had breakfast and still felt bleary-eyed and foggy, he wanted to get some fortification before the meeting started.

As he idly walked around the conference room, nursing a cup of black coffee and munching a massive apple fritter, Allan had to admit to himself, even in his dejected mood, that the surroundings were impressive. The oval table and the high-backed chairs with their gold brocade upholstering were standard fare. But the shelves full of first-edition, leather-bound medical books, somehow even the overly ornate mantel clock over the fireplace, gave the room a quiet and reassuring dignity. Maybe, he said to himself, summoning what little bit of wry humor was left within him, the others would understand this was no place to hold a kangaroo court.

They began to file in. Dorr came first, accompanied by his secretary who had brought a tape recorder and a fresh stenographer's notebook with her. Dorr shook hands with Allan, said a curt hello, then went to discuss recording procedures with his secretary. A man and a woman came in briskly, both carrying expensive leather attaché cases. Allan studied them, amused by their look-alike dress. The man, who was tall and heavyset, wore a severe, gray pin-striped suit, complete with vest. The woman, about five-foot-ten herself, Allan judged, had on a feminine equivalent of a man's business suit. Yet the man, with his well-styled hairdo and salt-and-pepper mustache, still managed to look a little more human than his companion, whose face, devoid of makeup, made her look like a department-store dummy waiting to be prepared for show.

Dorr looked up and rose to greet them. Allan could hear the woman say that they were Joyce Cole and Randolph Astor, the attorneys representing the University. They would be handling the defense against the artificial-blood lawsuit. Anthony and Harrison Cummings breezed in next, a jaunty spring to their steps, an attitude clearly meant to impart to those already present that they had the upper hand in the matters to be discussed. Jack White, the University hospital administrator, was the last to arrive. He nodded, said hellos, waved, but did not bother to take his turn of the room to shake hands with those who had already arrived. He pulled a chair away from one end of the table and sat down.

Taking their cue from him, the others, coffee, juice, or doughnut in hand, arranged themselves around the table. Allan withdrew to one of the chairs that stood against a side wall.

White cleared his throat, smiled thinly at Anthony and Cummings. "Shall we get started?"

Cummings and Anthony smiled back. If snakes could smile, Allan thought, cobras would smile like that.

"Before we go any further," said Joyce Cole, "I'd like to clarify just whom Mr. Cummings is representing. Is it Coit Hill Memorial, Harrison? Or the Gerbetti family?"

"The family, Joyce." Cummings stressed the woman's first name.

"Ah, the family. Then what, may I ask, is Mr. Anthony doing here?"

"I'm here as an interested party, ma'am. Young Gerbetti, after all, died at Coit Hill Memorial."

She ignored Anthony. "I have doubts about the propriety of this," she said to Cummings.

"I certainly appreciate your concern, Joyce," Cummings answered, enunciating every word. "If my standing in this, or Mr. Anthony's, is of concern to you, we can terminate at this point and rely on the usual procedures. It was the University's counsel that requested this meeting. I am here merely as a courtesy to a friend, one of your very own senior partners."

"I was merely—"

"Ladies and gentlemen?" White broke in. "We agreed that this was to be an informal discussion, an exploration of points we could agree on. Shall we try to keep it in that spirit?"

Cummings and the woman glared at each other, then looked away to the papers in front of them.

Anthony broke the ensuing silence. "Now, I'm not the lawyer, but from my point of view there are two issues here that we need to talk about." He stopped and looked around the table, as if daring someone to interrupt him, to challenge his version of matters. No one made an attempt.

"The first, and maybe the most important from our point of view, is the vendetta the University's agents have been carrying on against Coit Hill Memorial and the other community hospitals. Our reputation and our standing in the community have been adversely affected by—"

"What do you mean, 'agents'?" Allan interrupted.

Dorr, who had been sitting with his back to Allan, pivoted in his seat and fixed hard eyes on the young man. Allan did not continue.

"The second is the death of the Gerbetti boy in our emergency room as a result of the unauthorized use of a highly experimental procedure. That too has served to besmirch our reputation and has caused us severe damage."

"So that in sum, Mr. Anthony, what we are discussing here is not patients or patient care, but Coit Hill Memorial's sullied reputation?"

Allan leaned forward to make sure that it was Dorr who had spoken.

"Patient care, Dr. Dorr, depends as much on the value of a hospital's name as on anything else," Anthony said. "A hospital whose reputation suffers can't draw good physicians, donors of needed funds, can't provide the medical services that its patients need. It seems to me that a University physician, more than anyone else, Dr. Dorr, should be able to appreciate that."

White held up his right hand. "Look, this is getting us nowhere. Let's just put our cards on the table. What will it take to get this business cleared up, so that we can all go back to our work again?"

"Mr. White," Joyce Cole said before Anthony or Cummings could reply, "as the University's attorney, I must caution you against the way you are trying to rush this matter to completion. While we are interested in exploring the possibility of an amicable resolution, please bear in mind that the pending legal action—"

White sighed audibly. "What I am trying to do here, Ms. Cole, what we are trying to do here, is to see to it that there is no 'pending legal action.' It won't do the University any good and, Mr. Anthony's solid faith in his institution notwithstanding, it won't do Coit Hill Memorial any good to have this drag on, either in the newspapers or in the courts."

She looked at her partner, who, almost imperceptibly, shrugged his shoulders. She crossed her arms angrily and leaned back. "I'm not sure why you even asked the firm to send us," she said quietly as she took off the half-glasses she had perched toward the bottom of her nose. Allan wondered whether she wore them to make herself look older than she was.

"To consider the reputation of Coit Hill Memorial is all well and good," Cummings said. "But first let us talk about an only child, a young man who was well on his way to becoming a professional, the first in his family to go to college, the one to whom his parents could look for some promise of financial security when they retired—"

"Spare us, Cummings," Randolph Astor said. "What will it take to make the family whole?"

"In terms of bereavement, loss of income, mental anguish over losing their son, anguish over having him made into little more than an experimental animal . . ."

Astor leaned forward on the table. "Spare us the bullshit, Cummings. How much?"

"Three-point-five million dollars."

Cole shook her head as if her disbelief could not be expressed in words, then leaned forward, opened her files, and put on her glasses again. "I've checked the court calendar," she said to Astor. "We can get an early motion for summary judgment on September tenth."

"Fine with us, Joyce," Cummings countered. "But I doubt that by that time you would even have had time to answer our first interrogatories."

Dorr held up his hand, seeking recognition. "Mr. Cummings, as a physician and as an administrator here I'm keenly aware of malpractice settlements, so I don't believe I'm talking out of order. Surely you must realize that even by California standards, a three-and-a-half-million-dollar settlement is a trifle high."

"And what's the point, Harrison?" It was Astor. "Assume you reduce some jury to tears and get your award on the trial level. A trial judge isn't likely to let it stand at more than half of that and an appellate court most certainly isn't likely to. So if we're here to make a good-faith effort to settle this without a long, drawn-out fight, why gum things up with a preposterous figure like three and a half million?"

Cummings leaned forward and poured himself another cup of coffee from one of the thermos containers on the table. "In the first place, a settlement of three and a half million dollars is not unheard of. In the second place, there is no guarantee that either a trial judge or an appeals court is going to be moved to cut it. In the third place, you are ignoring the punitive damages I expect any jury to award under the circumstances of this case. But if you are serious, we'll accept your settlement offer of one-point-seven million right now."

"What settlement offer of one-point-seven million?" Cole asked.

"Why, I understood your partner to say that even under the most optimistic circumstances he can foresee your client should expect to be liable for one-point-seven million dollars. Naturally, I must presume that you'd be willing to settle for at least that much to avoid not only the attorney fees and court costs, but the publicity during the considerable length of time it will take to get to trial, not to mention any appeal your client may choose to pursue. We'll accept the one-point-seven million dollars."

"No such offer has been made, Cummings, and you know it," Astor huffed.

"Look, instead of sparring over momentarily meaningless numbers and wasting our time disagreeing, can we try to find some common ground, some things we can, at least for a start, agree on?" Dorr asked.

They all turned toward him. "First, in regard to the death of the boy, I think we can agree that, if at all possible, we should avoid a trial. To be blunt, it would be harmful to the University."

Anthony humphed.

Dorr trained his eyes on him. "Don't be so self-righteous, Mr. Anthony. You may get away with portraying Coit Memorial as a victim in all of this for about ten seconds. But the fact remains that in a trial it will become very apparent that Coit Memorial's responsibility could be just as great as the University's. It was, after all, your emergency room that hired Dr. Kirk. The University did not impose him on you."

Dorr held his breath. He had meant what he had said and had worded it sharply to stop Anthony. But he was afraid his remarks would set off Allan. No explosion came. And no one else found reason to contradict him either.

"So, then. Let's assume for the moment that without arm-wrestling over every detail, there is at least some agreement to make proper compensation to the Gerbetti family. Now, what else need we talk about?"

"What we need to talk about is why the University wants to gain a monopoly on all trauma cases in this county and damage the very fine service we are developing," Anthony said.

"Mr. Anthony, the University is trying no such thing."

"It isn't? It hasn't sent out one of its key physicians, someone who has just been appointed to a newly created department of trauma surgery, to raise hell all over the county about what terrible care trauma victims get at community hospitals?"

"No one has sent anyone on any kind of a mission."

"Then the best that can be said is that your Dr. Kirk is an unguided missile. And even there you're responsible. He's your missile. If you didn't rein him in, we must assume that he talked, if not with your authorization, then with your tacit approval."

"Again, I don't want to dwell on the negatives: that will get us nowhere. Mr. Anthony, the University is not anxious, has no interest, in denying you the ability to handle trauma cases. Let me just ask you simply. What would put your mind at ease—besides, of course, the University making an overt effort to abridge Dr. Kirk's constitutionally protected right to say what he believes?"

Anthony drummed the fingers of his right hand on the tabletop. "It seems to me," he began slowly, "that there are enough trauma cases in the San Francisco area to make everybody happy. I think we can work things out."

"What do you mean by that?" White asked.

"Let's come to an agreement. You people take all the cases that are within a three-mile radius of your hospital. And we'll take everything beyond that. Clean and simple."

"Mr. Anthony, you certainly are generous," White said.

"Most of the area around here is where the majority of the stabbings and shootings are. So what you're giving us are people who'll come in here with serious penetrating trauma and not one cent of coverage. And you get to go out and look for the car-accident people who are insured to the teeth. What an offer! And you know very well that without the county contract to treat the nonemergency patients we couldn't even handle the cases you are leaving to us. How are we going to staff even a modest trauma service?"

"Oh, well," Anthony said expansively. "If we were to be guaranteed a steady flow of trauma cases, why, we wouldn't even have time to undertake the contract we've been discussing with the county. No, we just couldn't handle both." He sat back, immensely satisfied with himself.

Dorr turned to White. "I don't like what Al is saying, but let's not be totally unrealistic about this. I think a payment on the boy's death is unavoidable. Being assured of getting the county contract renewed could give us some common ground on which we can de-emotionalize all this. And taking trauma cases from our immediate area could also be part of a workable solution. I think we're heading in the right direction. It will get us out of a difficult situation."

White studied Dorr. "I don't know, Phil. . . ."

"Well, at least we can think about it and then get together again to talk more," Dorr said, looking at his watch. "Right now, I've got another meeting to get to and I'm sure the others have a good deal to do as well."

Before Dorr could fully rise from his chair, Allan leapt out of his seat and pushed his way between Dorr and White. His face was ashen with anger, his neck muscles tight. Dorr, looking up in alarm, saw the artery along Allan's temple pulsating wildly. Allan erupted, his voice roaring.

"You bastards. You unprincipled, smug bastards. You sit around here crying crocodile tears for a dead kid, you talk millions of dollars like you're talking about last week's beef auction. There are people dying out there and you don't give a shit, you—"

Dorr held up his hand. "We've heard it all before. No one is interested. Nothing we can do will bring the boy back, so the least we can do is talk about a settlement for his family. And as for your trauma victims, they'll get help, Allan. Maybe not in the perfect way you want, but they'll get it."

"Where, Phil? In that schlock house that man calls a hospital? Do you honestly believe that? No one over there gives a rat's ass about trauma except Anthony and he only cares because he can jerk off while looking at the bills he'll submit to the insurance companies."

"Allan!"

Allan was now pacing furiously around the table. Cole shrank down into her seat, her partner stared dead ahead. Anthony watched Allan with glee, his eyes conveying the knowledge that he was watching a broken man in the final throes of his agony. White and Cummings merely looked at their hands.

"And what about me, goddamnit, what about me? You cut your little settlement deal on the kid, and what does that say about me? I'll tell you what it says. It says I fucked up, that I'm guilty, that I killed that kid. Who the hell gave you the right to do away with me that way? The artificial blood had nothing to do with that kid's death. Nothing. But if you settle this way, without fighting it, you're just helping the state get my license."

No one said a word. He looked around. No one would meet his gaze. Allan trained his eyes on Dorr, but even the older physician riveted his gaze on the shiny tabletop.

He didn't stop running until he had reached one of the several emergency exit doors on the hospital's first floor. The moment he pushed the long horizontal steel bar, the door's alarm shrieked, piercing the quiet of the hallway he had used to come this far. He ignored the wail and pushed so viciously at the door that it swung fully around on its hinges, crashing into the outside wall behind it. Allan bolted out and a half dozen steps from the exit, but, like a longtime convict who had engineered an escape plan but now was paralyzed by the need to choose a new direction to full freedom, he stood rooted to the spot. Angry, afraid, with no conception of what he could or should do next, Allan looked in every direction, even, for a moment, back to the hospital. When he shifted his eyes again, his gaze fell on a nearby bar, Dorothy's Tavern, which the hospital staff affectionately called "Dirty Dottie's." He made for the bar.

The conversation in the conference room began to seep back into his head and, as he heard each one of the participants repeat and repeat again the points of the proposed settlement, he grew angry again. He was so absorbed by his resentments that the touch on his arm only barely intruded on his thoughts. He turned to find Maggie Brooks walking along next to him. Allan guessed she had worked through the night because her greens were wrinkled and bloodstained. Her hair was tucked beneath a paper hat, but strands, sticky from sweat, stuck out. Her eyes were bloodshot and weary. Allan said nothing and kept walking.

"Where you headed?" There was a forced lightness in her voice.

"Dottie's."

"Little early in the day for that, isn't it?"

There was no response.

"Mind if I join you?" she asked, at the same time reaching into a pocket to make sure she had a beeper with her. "They probably still have some of yesterday's coffee on the burner and that's about the only thing that will keep me going for the last twelve hours of my shift."

Allan again remained silent. Doggedly, she kept pace with his seven-league strides.

"Someday, Allan, I'd like to take a normal, leisurely walk with you," she said, again trying to be casual by referring to their first marathon encounter some weeks back. "It'd be a whole new experience for both of us."

There was, again, no response as Allan stepped off the curb to cross the street.

He hadn't been in Dottie's in well over a year and a half. The moment he opened the door to be greeted by a cavernous dark gloom, he felt his skin crawl and remembered his aversion to the dingy, unkempt place. To his right was the bar. At 10:30 in the morning many of the stools were already occupied, including some taken up by men whom Allan recognized as regular visitors to the emergency room, men who either wandered in to sleep off a drunk in one of the reception-room chairs or who were carried in, hemorrhaging from stomach ulcers. Occupying the last stool at the far end of the bar was another regular, a mid-fiftyish, short, fat woman with a gigantic bouffant blonde wig. A cigarette dangled from her lips. She sat staring dead ahead, taking periodic, seemingly timed, swigs from the short glass in front of her.

To his left, and on the other side of the aisle, were the customary red booths, and Allan, followed by Maggie, made his way to one deep in the bar's interior. A large gold-on-black-velvet painting—a depiction of a bare-breasted young blonde sitting atop a bull—graced the wall above the booth. The lone waitress on duty slunk over, looked at Maggie and Allan, and waited.

"Scotch, a double," Allan ordered.

"I'll just have coffee," Maggie said after casting him a dubious look.

"It ain't fresh, honey," the waitress warned her.

"I know. Can you fix me a sandwich or cook up something?"

"Don't know if we have anything left, sweetie. Some roast beef, maybe."

"Good enough."

When the waitress left, Maggie put her hand on Allan's arm. "There's no sense being mad at me too, or, for that matter, at the rest of us."

"I'm not mad at you or the rest of you."

"There's talk of a residents' strike to protest what the University is doing to you. Those things aren't supposed to happen anymore, Allan. It's not fair and there are a lot of people who are really pissed."

"Why? Because they figure that if it can happen to me it can happen to them too?"

Maggie looked pained. "Allan . . ."

"I'm sorry." He softened somewhat. "I'm out of line. This isn't the sixties anymore. Hell, it's not even the seventies. You all go on strike, they'll fire you and have you replaced before you've had a chance to roll up your stethoscopes and put them in your pockets."

"But it's not fair!"

The waitress set Allan's drink in front of him, then put down Maggie's sandwich. Maggie carefully lifted the top slice of limp white bread as if she half expected some loathsome creature to come slithering out. There were two thin slices of roast beef, each slightly browned and curled around the edges. Mayonnaise covered the underside of the bread. She scraped the dressing off, squirted a healthy dose of mustard on the meat out of a stained and crusted plastic squeeze bottle, and replaced the bread. "Look out for the first signs of botulism, will you?" she asked as she prepared to take a first bite.

"Fair has nothing to do with it," Allan said. "When the University created the trauma surgery department, they looked on it as maybe another interesting little service they could provide, and maybe as another way of expanding their training program. They were just looking for something that would give the University some more sheen."

"Then why aren't they backing you?"

"Because they hadn't counted on trauma becoming a political issue. Because they are scared shitless of Anthony. Because, basically, they're gutless. When they face a tough fight, quality care becomes secondary to them." Allan had quickly finished his Scotch and signaled the waitress for another one. The waitress came over, put the drink down. He picked it up and took a long swallow.

"And you're going to do nothing?"

"Nothing." He lifted the tumbler, looked at the liquid in it, and took another drink. "Nothing at all."

Maggie tried hard to think of something that would spark a positive response in him. For days she and the other residents and interns had been speculating about his response to the misfortunes that had befallen him and there was no one who had even suggested that he would not fight back. His absence from the hospital, it had been widely rumored, was as much self-imposed as ordered. Over lunch, at coffee breaks, in the off times between emergencies, Maggie had heard that Allan, the fighter, Allan, the man who could always be counted on to do battle against the administrators in behalf of medicine, would be back soon, an invincible battle plan in hand. And yet here he was getting drunk, not only refusing to go on the offensive, but even refusing to put up much of a defence.

"Allan, we'll help. Maybe a strike isn't a good idea. But there is something we can do," she pleaded.

"How's the jogger?"

For a moment Maggie was confused by the sudden switch in the conversation, but she went along. "Fine; very well, in fact. We CAT-scanned him and found that the source of that damned infection was an abscess below the right lobe of the liver. We opened him up again, took out the twelfth rib, and put in a drainage tube. I'd say he's turned around. His lungs are clearing and we've got our fingers crossed on his kidneys. We still have him on dialysis but he's started to produce urine. Yesterday, for the first time, Fedder admitted that he might have a chance of making it."

"His wife?"

"Doing much better too, obviously." She stopped, then continued. "We've gotten to be good friends. I had dinner over her house the other night."

Allan polished off the drink. He had not had so much hard liquor in years and he could feel the effect it was having on him. He felt a faint buzzing throughout his body. He had the impression that he had somehow stepped out of the scene, that he was there observing himself and Maggie talking. For a few seconds he was transfixed by the feeling. He watched Maggie's mouth move without having the slightest notion of what she was saying. He called out to the waitress for a refill.

The feeling passed and he realized that he had not responded to Maggie's comment about her new relationship with the jogger's wife. "That's taking things a bit above and beyond the call, isn't it?"

She looked hurt.

"I didn't mean that as a criticism, Maggie. I was just teasing. If she invited you it's because she feels that you've helped her through."

"I hope I have."

"So emergency and trauma medicine aren't impersonal blind dates for you anymore?" For the first time Allan smiled.

"No, they're not blind dates anymore. I made up my mind about something. I've applied for a surgical residency next year. I want to do trauma."

"You're giving up psychiatry?"

"It's your fault, my friend. After being around the team and, well, to be honest, after seeing what you have done with people and what I could do, it just didn't seem like I should spend the rest of my life either with Marin County neurotics or, for that matter, San Francisco psychotics."

She waited. "No reaction?"

He managed another smile. "It's great, Maggie. You'll do good work. Hell, you're a warm person, you'll do great. Trauma needs people like you. Just don't . . . get involved with the system itself. Just your patients, Maggie, just your patients."

"So, why can't you follow your own advice." She stopped. "Sorry, that was stupid."

Allan drank and watched the woman in the bouffant hairdo struggle off her barstool. She stood behind it, then pushed herself away from the bar, as if pushing a small rowboat away from a dock. With a determined step she walked toward Allan and Maggie, then stopped. She looked at Maggie, then looked intensely at Allan. "What a nice boy," she announced, her voice coming from vocal chords that had been subjected to too many cigarettes and too much alcohol. She took a drag from the lighted cigarette in her hand. The effort made her waiver slightly. "A nice boy." She turned and went on her way, in the general direction of the bathroom.

Maggie stuffed the rest of the sandwich in her mouth and followed it with a last swig of coffee. "I have to go, Allan," she said after making a strong effort to swallow the large bite she had taken. "Look, I know it looks terrible, but everybody is pulling for you." She reached out to him. "I know I don't have to tell you something you already know, but we all owe you a lot. There isn't a person on that service you haven't gone out of your way to help professionally or personally. Give us a chance to help you now. Please."

Allan looked down into the nearly empty glass before him. "Thanks," he answered quietly. "Sure, I'll give you guys a call."

She looked at him, sorrow plainly etched in her weary face, then leaned over and kissed him on the cheek. "We love you, Allan, don't forget that."

He nodded, then, as Maggie hurried down the narrow aisle to the door, he waved his hand at the waitress and pointed at his glass.

When he staggered out of the bar it was nearly two in the afternoon. The intense sunlight striking his eyes after four hours in the bar and the weight of the liquor he had consumed struck him hard. He felt dizzy. He stumbled forward, holding his forearm above his eyes, trying to adjust to the sudden brilliance. He weaved his way down the sidewalk, not truly aware of where he was heading, not really caring. He remembered that his car was at the hospital and as he turned around to head back to retrieve it, his feet tangled and he stumbled to his knees. Slowly he got up, looked in the direction of the hospital, then turned and walked away. After an hour of wandering aimlessly through residential and business areas, he found another bar and, without giving the matter a second thought, turned in.

At the far end of the bar a man was bent over, his head resting on the bar. Two stools away a woman nursing a beer was watching an episode of one of the afternoon soap operas. There were only three tables in the rest of the bar and each one had four or five chairs, turned upside down, on it. Toward the back, under a dim yellow light, stood an old pool table, two cues, and three balls sitting on its surface.

The bartender, who, with his back to Allan, also had been watching the soap opera, now turned around. A dirty dish towel was tucked into his belt. His white shirt was yellow with age. Slowly, chewing a toothpick, he walked over to his new customer. Allan put a twenty-dollar bill on the counter. "Scotch. Till this is gone."

When the twenty dollars had disappeared, he careened out of the bar. Hunger gnawed at him. Trying to focus as he stumbled along the street, he looked for a place where he could buy something to eat. He managed to walk into a tiny Chinese restaurant and sat down at an oilcloth-covered table. A red-jacketed waiter came over, took the menu from between the sugar container and the paper-napkin holder, and handed it to Allan. In his befuddled state, his eyes fell first on the Chinese characters describing the available dishes. He was about to fly into a rage at the impassive man standing next to him when he finally managed to fix his eyes on the English portion of the menu. Even then he had a hard time reading the offerings because the words, when they were not dancing, were moving in and out of focus. He thought he saw beef in oyster sauce offered and ordered that and a bottle of beer.

When the waiter had placed his food in front of him, Allan reached for the paper-covered chopsticks next to the fork. Slowly, as if he were undoing a particularly beautiful gift-wrapping paper he did not want to destroy, Allan opened the envelope holding the sticks. When he had accomplished the task, he took out the chopsticks and, again moving slowly and deliberately, carefully broke the chopsticks apart. Concentrating, he gripped the utensils and aimed for his plate. As he maneuvered to pick up some of the beef, his fingers slipped. Half of the plate's contents spilled onto his lap. He tried again, this time bending close to the plate and narrowing his eyes to sharpen his focus. He managed to pick up two pieces of beef and brought them to his mouth. After half a dozen passes at the plate, he dropped the chopsticks and ran to the toilet. He was barely inside the door before the day's liquor and the few pieces of food he had managed to eat came up on him. He fell to his knees in front of the stained toilet bowl and vomited, until the spasms, though continuing to wrack his body, brought forth only thin, bitter bile.

He pushed himself off the floor and bent over the small washbowl. He turned on the single tap on the basin and splashed cold water on his face. He cupped his hands, took some water into them, and sipped it into his mouth. He rinsed, spat the water back out. As he passed his table, he dropped a ten-dollar bill on it and walked out.

He was tired, his legs ached, and his head throbbed, but he couldn't face returning to his apartment. He passed a movie box office, stopped, and turned back. Without bothering to look at the marquee and only noting on the ticket price list that the theater was open twenty-four hours, he took a five-dollar bill out of his pocket. He pushed it toward the cashier, but missed the small opening in the window. He tried again, now concentrating on his task, watching his hand as, trembling, it pushed the bill forward. The cashier, anxious to help him along, took hold of the fiver's corner and drew it toward her, then waved him through the turnstile at the side of the ticket booth. The lobby was deserted. Feeling a recurrence of his hunger, Allan staggered to the food counter. But the shelves, he saw, were devoid of candy. He turned to the popcorn machine and studied it extensively. It too was empty save for a few unpopped kernels and a scattering of popped corn on its rusted bottom.

The theater was dark and Allan kept his eyes on the floor, trying to find his way down the aisle to a seat in the middle of the auditorium. When he had chosen his row, he stumbled over a man who had staked out a spot on the aisle and moved to a middle seat. Once seated, he took off his tie and coat, leaned back in the seat, and only then looked up. He was greeted by a view of a gigantic penis, a woman's face on each side of the shaft, each woman bestowing her favors upon its owner. He was momentarily startled, but as the kissing and slurping continued, his eyelids closed and he fell asleep.

He woke up twice, once to a scene of a woman handcuffing a squirming man to a brass bed stand, then later to two female lovers wielding dildos on each other. But the third time he opened his eyes it was because a bony finger was tapping on his shoulder. He looked up to see an elderly, slightly stooped black man, holding a decrepit broom, standing next to him. "Come on, buddy," the man said. "Seven o'clock in the morning. You had your chance to sleep it off, now go on, get outta here." There was nothing friendly in his voice, nor in his eyes.

Allan looked around. Three other men were rousing themselves, apparently also because the janitor had woken them up. Slowly, his every muscle stiff and rebelling against the effort, Allan lifted himself from the seat and left the theater. He trembled when he looked around him in the street. The area was filled with small bars, porno shops, boarded-up windows. As he shuffled down the sidewalk, he passed men, some alone, some in groups of two or three, sitting on stoops, crouched in doorways, reclining against walls. He could feel their hostile looks as they, the regulars in the area, wondered who this new derelict was, why he had wound up among them.

When a cab cruised by, he hailed it. The taxi stopped, but when he went to open one of the back doors, he found it locked. The cabbie rolled open his window. "Show me your money first, buddy." On the verge of just allowing himself to collapse in a heap in the middle of the street, Allan rummaged around in his pockets. He found his last ten dollars. He also found the key to Julie's apartment, which she had given him in Napa. He gave the cabbie the ten dollars and Julie's address. The lock on the back door popped open, and Allan fell in.

He made his way slowly up the stairs, not quite sure why he was at the apartment, what he would say to Julie. Leaning against the door jamb, he rang the bell. There was no answer. He rang again. He looked at his watch. It was nearly eight and he remembered that she usually was out of her apartment and on the way to work by 7:30. He dug the key to her door out of his pocket and let himself in. He went into her bedroom and, without bothering to pull back the quilt covering the bed or taking off his shoes, he collapsed on the bed.

Returning from the medical examiner's office at a little before six that evening, Julie walked slowly up the stairs to her apartment. It had been a hard day, not only because work had piled up, but because she had not heard from Allan. She had called his apartment almost every hour, had even called the hospital half a dozen times, leaving messages, asking to have him paged. She tried desperately to think of a friend of his she could call. Allan had mentioned one or two people, but because he had not yet introduced her to any of his friends or colleagues, she knew no last names and didn't know whom to call.

When she reached the top of the stairs, she stopped. The door to her apartment was slightly ajar. She looked to the left of the landing, then to the right. She saw no one. Slowly, moving as quietly as she could, she turned around and tiptoed down the stairs. She knocked at the door of her neighbor on the lower level. There was no answer. She hurried out the front door and to the telephone booth at the corner. Because there had been two rapes in the neighborhood within the last month, some of the people who lived on the block had formed a Neighborhood Watch committee and had invited the commander from the local precinct to come and discuss safety precautions. She searched her memory for the phrase the officer had said they should use when calling if there was an emergency. Only as she was dialing the police department number did she remember. "This is a hot prowl," she told the police operator when he answered and quickly described what she had found. She was only halfway back to her apartment when the two patrol cars came to a screeching halt in front of the building.

She ran up to the cars as three policemen and a policewoman jumped out of the vehicles. All four unsnapped the leather straps holding their nightsticks and their guns.

"I'm the one who called," she told them quickly and again repeated the story of the rapes, of finding her door open. One of the policemen and the policewoman made their way to the rear of the building. The other two men, with Julie behind them, scurried up the steps to her apartment.

"Lady," one of them said brusquely, "keep out of the way, would you?"

She hesitated, then retreated halfway down the stairs, but not so far that she could no longer keep an eye on her door. The men, moving quietly and slowly, went to the door. They both drew their guns. One man moved to the left side of the door and put his hand on the doorknob. The other man stood off to the right. At a signal from the policeman on the right, the officer who had taken hold of the knob pushed the door open. Nothing happened.

Cautiously, they moved in. Julie moved up two steps. She saw them open her hall closet, close it, then turn toward her kitchen. She moved up another step. A second later she saw them head down the hall toward her bedroom. The sounds of shouting and scuffling forced her to retreat back two steps. And then she heard, in Allan's clear voice, "Goddamn sons of bitches," coming almost simultaneously with the single gunshot.

12

As she started to run up the five remaining steps, Julie tripped and fell. The fourth step slammed into her left kneecap, the top stair cut into her cheek. The edge of yet another step rammed into the heels of her hands as she tried to cushion her fall. Ignoring the sharp pains that flared through her, she picked herself up and, virtually on all fours, made her way to the landing leading to her door. She straightened out and barged into her apartment. She was barely inside the door before the police officers who had covered the rear of the building came storming in, pushing her aside. Stumbling as she tried to hurry, she followed them into her bedroom. Her scream on entering the room startled the four officers, now gathered around Allan's inert and spread-eagled body on the bed. A bloodstain was visible beneath and to the left of his head. Alerted by Julie's movements, the policewoman looked up in time to catch her as Julie lunged toward them.

"It's all right, lady, he can't hurt you. Just sit down and take it easy," the policewoman said, trying to assure her.

Wild with panic, Julie tried to free herself, tried to look around the woman's shoulder at Allan.

"Is he dead? Why did you have to shoot him?" she screamed. "Why did you have to shoot him?"

"Lady, the man broke into your apartment," one of the men said quietly. "If you had come in you could have been his third victim. In any case he's not—"

"Oh, my God, what have I done?" Julie sobbed as the policewoman gently guided her to the desk chair in the corner of her bedroom. "Allan . . ."

The three men still at the bedside stared at Julie. One of the men, the oldest among them said, "You know this guy?"

Julie said something, but her words were inaudible.

The older policeman crouched down. "Beg your pardon, ma'am?"

"He's my . . ."

"Boyfriend?"

"Yes," she whispered.

"And you didn't know he was here?"

"No."

"You didn't have a lover's quarrel before you called us?" one of the men asked.

Julie's eyes widened with fear as she grasped the implication of his question. "Are you out of your mind?"

The policewoman waved to quiet her colleagues. "Okay, let's take it easy here. Do you mind just telling us what's going on?"

Julie started to cry. "I don't know. Yes, I do. He's a doctor. He's been having trouble at the hospital where he works. When I last talked to him a couple of days ago he sounded terrible. I've been calling him every few minutes, at his apartment, at his office at the hospital. I haven't been able to get him. It just never occurred to me to call here today. He has a key, but he's never come here alone before. Never."

A groan came from the bed. Allan was stirring.

"In any case, he's far from dead," one of the policemen said. "When we came into the bedroom, he was asleep. I guess we took him by surprise. We tried to cuff him, but the minute I touched him he was on his feet, swinging. He took a kick at me and hit my hand. He was lucky my revolver was pointing down because the shot went into the floor. My buddy here let him have it with the nightstick."

Julie went over and helped Allan sit up. He groaned, put his hand to his head, and looked, perplexed, at the blood on his hand. Julie started to go to the kitchen to make an ice pack for him.

"Lady," the older man said, stopping her, "in the future, I'd be a little more careful with the 'hot prowl' call if I were you."

When the police officers had trooped out, Julie rummaged through her kitchen drawers until she found a plastic bag. As she was filling it with ice, Allan staggered in. His hair was badly disheveled, matted with blood, but also, it seemed to her, with sweat and dirt. His cheeks were covered by a two-day beard growth. His eyes were inflamed but dull, almost expressionless. Julie watched him, her emotions ricocheting within her. She was angry because he had excluded her from what were obviously agonizing and climactic events in his life. But then she suddenly found herself pitying him, despairing for his professional, personal, and emotional life. Then, just as quickly, the anger returned, fueled by her conviction that he had all too willingly and quickly adopted the role of the powerless victim.

Neither of them spoke. Allan sat down on one of the dinette-set chairs. Julie put a rubber band around the top of the now ice-laden plastic bag and then wrapped it in a dish towel. Wordlessly she handed it to Allan, who gently lowered it to the spot where the nightstick had caught him.

Julie didn't know where to start. "You want something to eat or drink?" she asked, deciding finally on the neutral topic of alimentation.

Allan just shook his head. Julie started to pour herself some wine, then decided she had better keep a clear head, and instead put water on the stove to make herself some tea. Allan, his head lowered so he could position the ice bag better on his wound, didn't make an effort to look up or talk.

Julie waited for the water to boil, then poured it into a mug. She put a tea bag in, then faced him. "Allan," she finally said, working to keep her voice steady. "Since we've been back from the trip we've had exactly one five-minute phone conversation. You don't call me, you don't answer your phone. I need to—"

"Julie, please don't. . . . I don't need another issue to contend with right now."

She drew back. "I'm sorry, Allan, I didn't realize that my asking to be part of your life would annoy you."

He picked up the ice bag and held it against his head again.

"Allan."

He said nothing.

"What are you going to do?"

"There is nothing to do. Let them do whatever they want. It's all irrelevant to me anyway."

"I'm not really sure I understand you. What do you mean it's all irrelevant?"

Allan slammed the ice bag against the table. The packet opened. Ice cubes and water flew in every direction. "It means exactly what it's supposed to mean. I'm on the verge of losing my license. I've got lawsuits coming at me from every side. The University is cutting itself a nice deal with the kid's family. They're admitting I'm guilty as hell and buying themselves out of the mess."

"And you're not going to fight?"

He leapt up, the chair flying backward and hitting the floor with a loud crash. "I am so sick of hearing that!" His voice took on a sarcastic whine. "'Aren't you going to fight? Aren't you going to fight?' Everybody's favorite question."

He came back to the table, put his hands on it, and leaned forward. "What am I going to fight? The University is not at all interested in contesting the artificial-blood suit. Dorr and White have all but offered to blow the kid's fag attorney to get a settlement."

"You could get your own lawyer," Julie said, trying to understand that he was under pressure, struggling to keep judgement out of her voice.

"Get my own attorney? Get my own attorney with what money? Do you have any idea what a malpractice suit costs to defend? I couldn't buy ten minutes of a good shyster's time. Don't you listen? If the University settles, they are as much as admitting that they're guilty, that I'm guilty."

"For starters, you could find a way of getting a lawyer. Go to the ACLU. Hell, I don't know what I would do, but at least I'd try to find out." Her frustration had cut loose her fury and she didn't try to hold herself back. "Have you even bothered to try to find out if an autopsy was done on the boy? Has anyone established that the artificial blood caused his death? You haven't even asked me to look to see if he was ever posted at the M.E.'s office. Has it occurred to you to try to find a pathologist who could help you? And if it's a question of money you know you can ask me."

"Why would I ask you? It's not your fight."

"I won't even dignify that with an answer. But I'll tell you something. You're making damned sure that it isn't your fight either. You don't want to fight. You've discovered this great truth about trauma care in this county and so you think that everybody should just drop dead with gratification and immediately solve the problem your way. Big surprise. They all have their own plans and don't much give a damn for yours. And you know what you're doing? You're acting like a child whose friends don't want to play according to his rules. You're just going to withdraw from the game. And you're too much of a fool to see that that isn't going to stop the game because it's not even your ball to take home out of spite. The game will go on, Allan, while you sink and drown in self-pity!"

"You're damned right I discovered something and damned right I think they should bust their butts to fix it. I've seen people bleed to death who should still be alive. And those people are dead because people like Anthony 'have their own plans.' And who the hell are you to preach to me? You sit in that office of yours at the M.E.'s office and reduce dying and deaths to meaningless statistics. As long as you can add up a thousand deaths and find out what the mean deviation is you're happier than a pig in shit. Don't talk to me about hiding from the realities of life."

They glared at each other. "Get out!" Julie finally said.

Allan turned on his heels and strode out of the apartment. Halfway down the stairs, he stopped, turned around, and went back up. From the threshold of the door, he flung the key to

Julie's apartment toward the kitchen. "Here you go," he called out viciously. "No need to spend another seventy-five cents to get another one made for the next guy."

The tall, middle-aged woman, whose light-sensitive glasses had not turned fully transparent even in the semidarkness of the cocktail lounge, extended her hand to Younger as he approached the table. The other, a younger woman, looked at Younger, but remained seated. A waiter approached and Younger ordered a double Scotch.

"Still trying to make trouble, Sam?" the middle-aged woman asked, but in a light tone.

"Only when I have to, Anna. Are you going to introduce me?"

"No, that's ground-rule one. Another one is that this is off the record. You can't use what we tell you, not unless you can corroborate and attribute it independently."

"Tough rules."

"Well, this is a young kid who can't afford to get fired, this is her first year out of school. She was working E.R. the night the mayor was at Coit Hill. It wouldn't take Al Anthony long to trace a story back to her."

"All right," Younger said. "Let's talk. What have you got?"

The woman turned to the young nurse. "Tell Sam what you told me."

"I was working with the night nursing supervisor, Miss Cluny, the night the mayor came in. About two in the morning, after the mayor died, Dr. Huntington came back to the emergency room. He was really upset. It was so odd, the way he was acting. He was turning everything upside down, trying to get together all the mayor's records, the lab studies, the nursing notes. He made a big fuss because the X-ray report wasn't back and available. He even went off to the X-ray department to look for it. After I came in for my next shift I was going through the interdepartmental deliveries. The X-ray report was there. I was curious so I looked at it. Then I gave it to Cluny, who immediately called Dr. Huntington."

"What did the X-ray report show?" Younger asked.

"It showed that the mayor had a right pneumothorax. At the time I didn't feel right about the whole thing, but I didn't know what to do and I didn't really have anyone I thought I could talk to."

Younger looked at the older woman. "There was no mention of a pneumothorax in the official report." He turned back to the younger woman. "Is there anyone who can substantiate that?"

"Only Miss Cluny," the young nurse said. "Or Dr. Huntington."

Younger left the two women and, since it was only 8:15, decided to go by Julie's apartment. He had not had a chance to talk to her since their first encounter. If Younger had harbored hopes that by now Allan would be back in her arms, it was a hope that dissolved when she answered the door. Julie was even more distraught than she had been when he first located her.

"You haven't seen Kirk," Younger said, stepping into the apartment and following her to the kitchen.

"Briefly. He was here. We had a fight and he stormed out."

"Where do you think he might have gone? Do you have any idea at all?"

She shook her head. "At this point I'm not very interested in looking for Allan. You want to find him, find him yourself."

Younger studied her, trying to think why she would suddenly be so lethargic about finding her friend. "Julie, we have to find him. The woman I called from here gave pretty good reason to think Coit Hill is covering up something in the mayor's death. I need him to see if there are ways we can track down the evidence. But, maybe more important, knowing that there might be a cover-up and being able to help prove it might help him too."

"Look. As I said, I'm not very interested in finding him. He may be a marvelous surgeon, but he's not going to win any prizes for sensitivity."

"I don't want to interfere in your personal affairs," Younger said slowly, "but you've got someone on your hands who's teetering on an edge. When you come down to it, this is a naïve kid who sees medicine in very simplistic, idealized terms. He's not capable of dealing with medicine's economic or political sides, and now the one thing that was the most important thing in his life has been destroyed. At this point he's not rational and he's likely to do something dangerous or silly. And no matter how you feel now, you wouldn't want anything on your conscience."

Julie looked up sharply. The image of a small car careening down a narrow road flashed through her mind.

"Are you okay?" Younger asked.

"Yes," she said, coming out of her thoughts. She added, softly, "I'll do what I can."

Julie walked around the apartment, gathering a coat, her keys, a wallet. "Let me ask you something," Younger said as he watched her make her preparations. "Has Kirk tried to do anything at all to fight this? Has he got an attorney? Any experts who can help him prepare a defense?"

Julie grimaced. "No, he's making all sorts of excuses. He says that it's a lost cause, that he doesn't have enough money. . . . "

Younger searched his coat for his notebook and a pen. He scribbled something on a page, tore it out, and handed it to her. "Tell him to give these guys a call, they'll be more than glad to help."

Julie studied the names as she closed the apartment door behind her. "Who are they?"

"Well, maybe except for Kirk, Roger Steinhardt is the last of the righteous people."

Julie cast him a quizzical look. "I mean that about Kirk," Younger said. "In any case, Steinhardt has made a lifelong specialty of defending unpopular clients and espousing even more unpopular causes. In the mid-sixties, when he was just barely out of law school, he bludgeoned the University of California into readmitting student radicals who had been suspended for making a lot of antiwar noise and agitating against the administration. For a while he was the lefties' darling, until they pressured the University to cancel a speech by a leader of the American Nazi Party. Good old Roger went to court and got an order telling the University it had to allow the speech and ordering the radicals not to interfere with little Hitler's appearance on campus. A year later Steinhardt defended two of the radicals who had been indicted for refusing to register for the draft and took their cases free of charge because their families, staunchly Republican and in favor of the Vietnam war, would not pay for their defense."

"A lot of people were committed like that once."

"Sure, but some of those people, many of whom were Roger's friends, are now in prestigious legal firms, corporate law departments, and even federal and state agencies. Not Steinhardt. He's still working out of a one-room office near an Oakland ghetto. Two years ago he filed a dozen police brutality cases against the city of Richmond and campaigned for a grand jury investigation of its police department. Last year he negotiated the closing of a toxic chemical dump next to a lower-middle-class neighborhood and won substantial out-of-court settlements that allowed the dozen or so families to buy homes elsewhere."

"So he'll help Allan because right now he's an underdog?" she asked as they reached the door to the street.

"That and because he owes me. About eight months ago I was investigating a rumor that doctors who deliver Hispanic babies at the county hospital were forcing the mothers to accept sterilization while they were still in the delivery room. I got pulled off the story because the paper needed me for other stuff and when it got to look as if I wouldn't get back on the sterilization story for a while, I turned what I had over to Steinhardt because I'd gotten to know him. He used my material to threaten a suit against the county of San Francisco in behalf of a dozen Hispanic women, got a good settlement, and got a couple of the doctors severely reprimanded."

She shook her head. "Is that how you survive? By trading information and favors?"

"Not all the time; but it helps. If information were a bank credit card, it would have almost an unlimited charge ceiling."

She looked at the slip of paper in her hand again. "And this other man, Walter Creighton? Does he owe you too?"

Younger laughed. "No, but he thinks he does. Creighton is a gentlemanly old scholar who somehow wound up being a pathologist. A few years ago I did a long profile about him for a national magazine. I guess it got him a lot of lay attention for the first time in his life. Because I mentioned some fairly interesting murder cases he had worked on, the article even got him guest appearances on television shows. He feels I helped him enjoy a little good notoriety and he's always been really helpful to me since." Younger looked at his watch. "I'm going back to the office to type up some notes in case I have to get a story going. But I'll check back with you about eleven or eleven-thirty."

"That's fine."

"Good. Get going and find our young hero."

Julie watched Younger walk briskly away, then turned to go to her car. She thought again of the road on Twin Peaks, of Allan, his face taut, charging out of her apartment and barreling down the stairs, and felt a shiver shake her.

13

Although the night watchman at the medical examiner's building assured Julie he had not let Allan in, the old man escorted her to the file room to make sure that Allan had not gained access before the building had closed at five. The room was dark. Julie flipped on the lights and made a quick tour of the tables and the aisles between the file stacks. There was nothing out of place, no sign that Allan had come to work here. She gave the night watchman her home phone number, asked him to call her if Allan showed up, and ran out of the building.

As she drove slowly out of the parking lot, a deep sense of frustration washed over her. Since she had known Allan, they had spent most of their time in the medical examiner's office or in one of their apartments. How could she possibly know where to look? Frustration gave way to depression as she passed the Mexican deli where they had eaten lunch the first day he came to talk to her. She slammed on her brakes and threw the car into reverse. The dining room was crowded, but Allan was not at any of the tables. This is not a late-night movie, she reminded herself. The hero has not gone back to the table where you two first met in the hope that you would come looking for him there.

She was driving along Marina Boulevard when the thought struck her. Watching her side and rearview mirrors constantly to keep an eye out for police cars, she sped onto Highway 101 toward the Golden Gate Bridge. At Lincoln she turned off and raced along the boulevard until it turned into El Camino del Mar. She slapped the steering wheel angrily with her hand, remembering that Geary or California would have given her faster access to her destination. Now she was forced to make her way through a largely residential area until she finally arrived at Sutro Heights.

The massive rocks far below the palisades, Allan had told Julie, were his "thinking place." When he felt low, when he had a hard problem to solve, he would wind his way down one of the paths leading from the parking lot to the cove. From there, if the tide were low, he sometimes walked out to the larger rocks, found one he could sit on, and then watched the seals on the boulders farther out in the ocean. The utterly abandoned way in which the sea creatures lounged under the rays of the sun induced a languor in him that, in time, allowed him to break through whatever emotional anxieties or intellectual blocks were hampering him.

She pulled into the lot and jumped out of the car. The night was warm, making the tangy ocean air bearable. The smell of salt tingled through her nostrils and, far below, she heard the slapping of the waves. The serenity of the Heights calmed her for a moment. But she remembered why she was here and looked around. Four other cars were in the parking lot and in the light of the moon she could make out entangled couples in three of the cars, all discreetly parked far apart. The fourth car was Allan's.

She peered into the automobile. Allan's white lab coat lay crumpled in the front seat. The backseat was empty. She ran toward the protective fieldstone wall, leaned on it, and peered over. But even with the help of the moonlight, it was difficult to make out whether the shape she saw far below her and a good thirty feet from shore was a seal, a human being in repose, or just a piece of rock worn by the elements into graceful curves.

She ran back to her car, took a flashlight out of her glove compartment, and ran to one of the openings in the wall from which several narrow, unofficial paths ran down to the ocean. Tripping and skidding, she made her way down the sharp incline, maneuvering to pass around large boulders, to step on or over the smaller ones. Halfway down she paused, aimed her flashlight below her, hoping that she would now be able to determine if Allan was down there. The sounds of the surf were stronger now, the playful lapping of the water yielding more and more to the sound of waves crashing against stone. She could feel her heart racing as she started walking, trying to place her feet on the more stable and solid areas in the path. Yet, for all her caution, the knee she had injured during Allan's confrontation with the police began to throb. As she neared the bottom, the path grew especially steep and she slipped, landing hard on her rear end. In trying to cushion her fall she automatically put her hand down, tearing away the scab that had formed after her fall on the stairs. She picked herself up and, shaking her hand, finished her descent. As she moved toward the water's edge, she swept the flashlight beam back and forth.

Allan was sitting on a large rock about twenty-five feet from shore, his back propped against an outcropping on the large boulder. From the way his head angled backward, Julie guessed that he had had fallen asleep. Water surrounded his perch, and a low wave that came sweeping up skimmed over it. The wave broke just in front of her, engulfing her feet in cold water. She watched as the water receded, first from the beach, then from around Allan's resting place.

"Allan," she yelled. "Please come back!"

He did not respond.

A larger wave came in. A portion of the rushing tide crashed against the rocks surrounding Allan, sending solid water and white spray high in the air. The rest of the wave came to her. She did not move, and the water scurried past her, losing its momentum only when it had gone a foot or two beyond her. She felt the drag of the water as it was now pulled back to the ocean to become part of the next wave, only to push farther and farther into the beach.

"Please, Allan. Wake up!"

The next incoming wave formed, assaulted the rocks, and made its powerful swipe at the beach. Julie waited for the moment that she could first feel the water pull back. As soon as it began its retreat, she followed it out. Pebbles and small rocks cut and pressed into her soaking sneakers as she tried to find footing in the wet and giving sand. Another wave now prepared its onslaught, and, as the water rose and broke over the stark stone, Julie jumped on to a large boulder. Cold water sprayed across her face, the taste of brine suffused her lips. Her clothes pressed wet against her body. She waited for the ocean to move back once again.

She spotted a boulder that was large and flat and jumped on it, forcing her feet flat against the slippery ledge it provided. Flashing her light again, she quickly located him, then ran the light back toward her slowly in order to survey the area between her and his reclining figure. There were three rocks between her and Allan. The one closest to her was only a few inches below her feet. The one ahead of it, however, was substantially lower; and the third one was nearly level with the water's surface. From where she stood, the gap between that last rock and Allan's seemed to be about ten feet.

Taking a deep breath, she leaped to the next rock. A wave crashed, spewing more water on her. She shivered in the slight breeze. When she was sure the water was moving back out, she jumped to the second rock and, almost without pausing, to the third one. A massive wave obliterated her yell for him, at the same time cascading water over her. She shone her light toward him but from her new vantage point could see only a part of him. As the water raced back toward the horizon, she began to move off her rock, hoping to make it across to him. She stopped because, on looking down to determine her footing, she saw that between her and Allan the bottom dropped off precipitously. If she stepped down onto the sand the next incoming wave could very well be over her head.

Even as she agonized, a wave, its white crest rolling and breaking downward, broke over a rock just ahead and to the left of Allan. The slap of the impact made her heart jump. Water broke in every direction, some of it disintegrating into a mist over Allan, the rest of it rushing past her, only a foot or two below the ledge.

She looked around in desperation. Then she knelt, pulled off one of her shoes, and hurled it toward Allan. It sailed past him and disappeared into the dark. She raised her other foot and took off the remaining shoe. She aimed carefully, then let go. The shoe struck him. Julie saw him bolt upright.

"Allan!!"

He looked around, disoriented, stupefied by the roar of the ocean, the light that was shining in his face, the call of his name. A new wave approached and crashed over him. Distraught, unable to move forward, unwilling to move back, Julie could only scream. When water had cleared the rock, she saw that he had been swept sideways off his perch but had somehow managed to grab onto a smaller boulder to the side. The next wave would engulf him completely, she was sure, and would send him crashing into the sharp edges of stone protruding through the water. Water was now near the top of her rock. She turned toward shore and yelled for help, for someone to bring a rope. She thought of the people far up above them, making love, intent on their passion, the windows of their cars shut tight against her pleas, and found herself close to tears.

She turned back and saw that he had managed to find a grip on the rock where he had been. Clenching her fists, she watched as he slowly hoisted himself, bringing up first one leg, then the other. For a moment, his head drooping forward, his back heaving up and down, he stayed still on his hands and knees as he drew breath deep into his lungs. Allan took a final gulp of air, then, fastening his hands on the narrow portions of the rock, he carefully stood up. He had barely made it to his feet before the next rush of the ocean swept over the rock, engulfing his legs in water.

She saw him stare into the glare of her flashlight and turn to where she was standing.

"Julie?"

"Yes, damnit!" Her voice broke and she waited before going on. "Can you make it back?"

Before he had a chance to answer, another wave hurled itself at him, then at her. Water cascaded everywhere. Julie instinctively closed her eyes and turned away as the stinging water pelted every inch of her body. When she opened her eyes and turned back, he had disappeared from view. She was about to dive in to look for him when she saw him clinging to his rock but on the side that faced her. Because the tide was high now, when the ocean moved away from them between waves, water remained between the rocks where the two of them were now isolated.

She fell to her knees. "What can I do? We have to get back to shore!"

"After the next wave comes in . . ." He paused to take in air. "I'll make a try for it when the backflow has stopped."

Almost as he finished speaking, she could see the foam of the coming wave begin to form. Torrents of water assaulted the rocks, passing over the surfaces glistening in the faint moonlight. Julie felt water pouring over her feet, spray pelting her face. She was shivering. She opened her eyes quickly and saw Allan twisting and turning as the remnant of the churning water moved past him. Crouching down, she watched the water carefully. For a moment the water seemed strangely paralyzed, only an eddy here and there marring its calm. Then, as if in answer to a signal, the water began to retreat, first slowly, then faster and faster. Keeping her flashlight on him she could see him struggling to hold on, to resist the powerful waters tugging his body with them. For another instant the ocean was still again; he pushed off. With furious strokes he headed toward her. He swam toward the middle of the rock where the boulder made a gentle descent toward the water. Julie moved back, lay on her stomach. Trying to ignore the sharp surfaces of the rock jabbing through her clothes, the cold sting of the water, she reached down. He grasped her hands and pulled himself halfway out of the water, then let go of one of her hands to take hold of an outcropping.

Another wave assaulted them. She could feel his hand slip in hers but, using her other free hand, she grabbed for his wrist and held on. The water passed, and he scurried up the rest of the way. She stood up and they collapsed into each other's arms, her breath coming in sobs, his in short, shallow gasps.

They clung to each other, Julie's arms tightly wound around Allan's neck, his hands squeezing her waist. Breathing a bit slower, he pushed her away and scrutinized her face.

"You all right?" he asked.

Her upper teeth clamped on her lower lip, Julie responded with only a nod of her head. Allan pulled her to him. "Hey, come on," he said softly. "It's over. It's okay."

She freed herself and looked intently at his face. It was, to her amazement, relaxed, calm. His eyes were sparkling. "I'm going to beat them too, Julie," he said. "I can beat those sons of bitches."

Spray from a breaking wave sprinkled over them.

She pushed herself up on her toes and kissed him lightly on his lips. "Come on," she said quietly, turning toward shore. "We'd better make a break for it."

He turned her to face him. "Julie, this may be the most understated thing I've ever said, but thanks for being here."

Steam rose slowly from the bathtub. Allan was submerged to his chin, his head resting against the tub's edge. Julie, sitting across from him, was cupping water into her hands and pouring it over her head and shoulders.

"I don't think I'm ever going to get out of this tub," Allan said, reaching for the faucet to let more hot water pour in. "God, that ocean was cold."

Julie reached for the bottle of brandy she had placed on a small table next to the tub and poured some into two snifters. She handed one to Allan. "You could have killed yourself out there."

Allan sat up and took a sip. "That's not why I was out there."

She said nothing.

"I didn't know what else to do," he went on. "I got a block away from your apartment and I realized what I had done. I wanted to come back, to apologize. But I couldn't. Not because I couldn't say 'I'm sorry,' but because I was so ashamed. Then everything hit me again. The University had cut me off, I was in trouble with every medical authority in the land, I was being sued by every trauma patient I had ever worked on, and I had just made sure that I had lost you. Julie, I've never been so low in my life. I just wanted to think, to try to find a way back."

Allan reached out to put the drink back on the table. He turned on both faucets and played them until the water coming from the spigot was lukewarm. He caught the water in his hands then splashed into his eyes, which were still burning from the ocean's salt. "You were right, you know," Allan said. "That was the thing that really made me mad."

"That I was right?"

"Not the fact that you were right, but what you were right about. I did want everyone to concede that my perception of the trauma problem was right and that everything had to be changed. And when no one wanted to go along with me, I turned into a five-year-old."

Moving her leg back and forth, Julie ran her toes lightly along the calf and shin of Allan's right leg. "Throwing tantrums isn't going to accomplish anything," she said. "That's all I was trying to tell you."

"I know, I finally realized that." Allan bolted upright. "But goddamnit, they drive you to that. They're so self-righteous in their defense of the system—"

"And you are not being self-righteous in the way you condemn them?"

"Maybe I am. But, damnit, I've got . . . I don't know . . . *good* on my side."

She laughed.

"I mean it, Julie. Listen, at one point I turned the television on and happened to catch an interview with a bigwig at Coit Hill. When I was fighting Anthony, I saw red all the time because I was convinced that the battle was just about economics, about making bucks for the hospital. But listening to that guy on TV, I really understood for the first time that there is something involved beyond money. You should have heard him. He was talking about Coit Hill with reverent words like it was some cathedral. The fine institution this, the fine institution that. He never mentioned patients, or disease, or death. Not once did he talk about human suffering or what role the hospital could play in alleviating that suffering. Listening to him, you just imagined virginal equipment, clean rooms with well-made and untouched beds, gleaming operating rooms. And not one patient around. I started fantasizing while he was talking. I could see him and the rest of the board of directors, all of them dressed in long white robes, walking slowly behind Anthony as he led them on a tour of veneration through Coit Hill. I . . ."

Allan stopped, suddenly aware that Julie's toes were now stroking the inside of his thigh and that with each caress they were moving higher and higher.

"You're not listening," he laughed.

"I am. I am." Splashing water, she maneuvered herself toward him. "It's nice to have you back and excited again."

Allan put his hands behind her head and brought her toward him. As they kissed, her hands stroked him and he drew nearer to her.

"This is impossible, Julie. We'll drown."

"No," she whispered, raising herself to a crouch, then turning around and lowering herself to her knees so that she was facing away from him. "Let's do it this way. Quickly."

Pushing himself away from the back of the tub, Allan moved toward her. Her sore knee rebelled and she lifted it off the bottom of the tub. But by holding onto the side of the tub, Julie managed to support herself as Allan established their rhythm. He placed one arm around her waist to give her more support. With the other hand he caressed her neck, her shoulders, her breasts. Their pace quickened. Water sloshed over the sides of the tub. Julie's hand slipped off the tub rim and they almost collapsed into the water. Undaunted, Julie regained her balance, pushed her buttocks back toward Allan. He bent forward. "I love you, Julie," he said. "I love you." He was repeating the phrase even as he felt himself and Julie surge toward climax.

The doorbell rang as they were drying each other off. Slipping into a bathrobe, Julie went to answer it; only when she opened the door did she remember that Younger had said he might stop by again. Before the reporter had a chance to step inside or say anything, she stepped out into the hall, partially closing the door behind her.

"Did you find him?"

"Yes, he was down at Seal Rock, thinking things over."

"Can I come in? I know it's late."

Julie hesitated and Younger caught the ambivalence. "You sure he's here?"

"He's here. It's just that . . ."

"He's too drunk to talk?"

"No! He's been through an awful lot and he needs some breathing room. Give us a couple of days."

She sensed the door open behind her and simultaneously saw Younger look past her shoulder. Allan, wrapped in a large bath towel, was behind her.

"Don't you think you've done—" Allan began, the memory of Younger's stories welling up.

"Allan," Julie interrupted and quickly told him about the woman in the nurse's association Younger had called and about the pathologist and the attorney the reporter had suggested would be of help to Allan.

"Look, I think we need to talk some more, but I can come back in the morning," Younger added.

"Never mind," Allan said, though his voice still carried an edge. "As long as you are here, come on in."

Younger looked at Julie. She nodded assent and led them into the kitchen. While Younger took off his jacket and Allan concentrated on making his towel more secure around him, she boiled water for tea.

"Well?" Allan finally asked.

Younger recounted his meeting with the two nurses in greater detail. "After Julie went off to look for you I was going to go back to the office," Younger went on, "but I decided to stop by Coit Hill on the way in case Huntington was there. He was. He couldn't elude me, so he agreed to talk some."

"Did you really think you could get anything out of him about the missing X ray?" Allan asked.

"Not really, but who knows, people always surprise me." Younger took a sip from his cup. "For the first fifteen minutes I just played it as if I wanted to include the mayor's experience in a larger story about the potential problems hospitals face when they have to give emergency medical treatment to political figures. Huntington was very self-possessed. He talked about the medical care the Kennedys got after their assassinations and the care Reagan got after the attempt on his life. Compared it all to the 'wonderful effort this hospital provided the mayor.' I let him go on," Younger said. "Now listen to this."

He took his tape recorder out of his pocket and fiddled with the rewind and forward buttons until Huntington's voice came on, saying, "and the mayor wouldn't have gotten better care if he had been taken to George Washington University like Reagan. Given the mayor's heart condition we did exceedingly well keeping him alive even as long as we did."

There were some shuffling noises on the tape. "The talk is, Dr. Huntington, that the mayor also suffered a pneumothorax and that the fact was not made public," Younger's voice said.

There was a second of quiet on the tape. "That's pure bullshit, mister," Huntington's voice said. There was another momentary silence. "If you'll excuse me," Huntington went on, "I have some sick patients who need attention."

"There was no injury to the lung?" Younger's voice persisted.

"I already said there wasn't. Don't waste my time on a ridiculous fishing expedition like that." There was a scraping sound, as of chair legs being moved on the floor. "Please excuse me."

"Okay," Younger's voice said, above a noise of paper crackling and other background sounds. "But if you ever want to talk about it, give me a call. Here are my office and home phone numbers."

Huntington laughed.

"Well, it may be funny now, doctor," Younger's voice said. "But sooner or later it won't be. This business is likely to come crashing down. Maybe you should start thinking about whether you are going to come down with it or whether you can salvage something out of it."

"I don't know what you are talking about," Huntington said.

"Fine," Younger said, "have it your way. But let me leave you with something else. If you do know something but don't want to give it to me, at least consider talking to Allan Kirk."

Younger pushed down on the Off button and looked up at Allan and Julie. "I have to hand it to him," he said. "He was very cool about it. You had to be watching him really carefully to see the twitch in his face when I mentioned the pneumothorax."

"What was that business about Huntington talking to me?" Allan asked.

"I'm sure, given his reaction, that he does know something but I'm also pretty sure he won't come to me. On the other hand,

I thought it worth mentioning your name because he might see you as an acceptable way of blowing the whistle. Maybe he'll figure that any information he has will at least help you."

"That's nice of you," Allan said. "In a sense, though, the mayor's death, if he did die of a treatable injury, is almost a secondary issue."

"A secondary issue? How?"

"In the sense that it is not important just because he is the mayor. It is relevant only in that his death is no different from a lot of deaths in this county. Whether he could have been saved or not, there are a lot of other people who could survive their injuries and do not."

Annoyance crossed Younger's face. "You've been saying that for weeks, Dr. Kirk. It's becoming an old refrain, even for me."

Blood rushed to Allan's face, but Julie reached out and put her hand on his.

"It's not that I don't believe you," Younger went on, oblivious to the storm that had just been aborted. "I think your suspicions are right on. But proving them is something else."

"I can prove they are more than suspicions."

Younger stared hard at Allan. "How?"

"Julie and I have been working on a study. We dug through the M.E.'s files and found one hundred trauma deaths that have occurred in hospitals. If you analyze what was done for the patients in each of the cases in the emergency room, how long it took to get them into the O.R., if in fact, they did make it to the O.R., and if you look at the amount of time it took for surgical consultants to come in, you can't escape the conclusion that at least forty-five of them died because they did not get the proper care."

"You're saying that forty-five out of a hundred trauma patients that come to Coit Hill die because the hospital can't get anyone to treat them?"

"No, no. That's the whole point. It's not just Coit Hill where screwups are taking place. They're happening in virtually every community hospital in the county. The one hundred cases and the forty-five deaths include patients from almost every hospital in this area. That's why I'm saying that there is a problem that needs to be addressed whatever we find out about the mayor."

Younger was looking at him expectantly. "What I'm saying," Allan went on, "is that just proving that the mayor's case was mishandled at Coit Hill won't accomplish much. Okay, Anthony's ass would wind up in a sling, the hospital and some of the docs would be in hot water, Coit Hill might even lose its accreditation. But that wouldn't change the system. Even if Coit Hill were to be shut down and boarded up, ambulances would still be taking patients to other hospitals and almost half those people would go on dying, needlessly, at those institutions. It's the whole system that needs to be addressed."

Julie repressed a smile. Now she was convinced beyond a doubt she had the old Allan back.

"Will you make the study available to me?"

Allan looked at Julie.

"It's up to you," she said.

"Two months ago, a month ago, I would have. But now I'm not sure. Not that I don't believe in the analysis Julie and I have done, but now I think I have to do everything I can to give it credibility that will allow it to stand up. I was hoping to take the raw data to three or four other trauma surgeons who would look at it and evaluate it independently and then find a way of releasing it so that it doesn't look like a publicity stunt."

"And how long do you think that would take?"

"I have no way of knowing. Three weeks, a couple of months maybe, given how busy the people are whom I want to bring into this."

Younger laughed. "Two months? Then you might as well forget it. In that time Anthony will have consolidated his position so strongly that nothing would change the situation. If you have any hopes of having an impact with the study, you have to go with it now."

"Sam, I've got no credibility left in this town. If I release the study now, the hospital council, Anthony, even the E.R. docs at the other hospitals would have it shot out of the water before noon."

Julie and the two men sipped at their tea. After a minute or two Younger spoke up. "All right, let's do this. Copy whatever records you have and give them to me. I know a couple of trauma surgeons down in the L.A. area who are pretty good at responding to things like this. I'll fly the records down in the morning and get them to go over them. If they confirm your conclusions, I can still get a story into Sunday's paper."

"They'd move that fast for you?" Allan asked.

"Yes."

Allan said nothing. Younger guessed he was wrestling with himself, trying to decide whether to give him the study or hold on to it in the hope that its publication in a medical journal would help rehabilitate him in the medical community's eyes.

"It's not a fair-trade off, Allan, but there it is. You can give me the study and let it have its immediate impact on the situation here. Or you can wait, publish in the New England Journal of Medicine and get some polite handclapping from your peers, but in the meantime give Anthony the time he needs to establish his bastardized trauma system."

Allan took a deep breath. "All right. Go ahead. Print the sucker."

14

The ten-year-old boy, taking advantage of the rapidly waning daylight hours of a Saturday evening in late summer, was racing his bike around the block.

"Hey, Bobby! Come on in and take your bath," his father yelled from the doorway. "You've already taken one spill today. That's enough!"

The boy lifted his racing bike hat off his head, loosening a mop of brown hair, and waved the hat at his father as he sped by. "Last lap, Dad," he called back. "I've got the world record in my pocket."

"That and half the dirt in the neighborhood," the man said under his breath, letting the screen door slam behind him as he returned to the house.

When he rounded the corner the boy lifted himself off the bike seat and began peddling even more furiously, the loose laces of one shoe slapping against the chain guard, his right knee peeking in and out of the massive tear in his jeans with every upward and downward stroke of his leg. He was the bicycle racer who, in the last minutes of a world championship, was sweeping, to the cheers of hundreds in the velodrome stands, to a world's record.

He turned a second corner, then a third, his speed even now picking up. As he rounded the fourth corner and began barreling down the sidewalk that would take him to the finish line far down the block—actually the row of red bricks that delineated the boundary between the lawn and the driveway at his home—he bent forward over the handlebars so that he could concentrate better on his goal. Thus he did not see, much less have a chance to avoid, the car as it made a sweeping and rapid turn into one of the driveways on his race route.

The boy crossed the driveway just as the car pulled in. Though the car's teenage driver slammed down hard on the brakes, the impact sent the little boy and the bike crashing into the closed garage door at the end of the driveway. The bike, crushed and twisted, slid down the garage door and came to a rest at the door's bottom. The boy bounced halfway back to the car.

While the teenager's parents frantically telephoned first for help, then to alert the boy's family, the teenager, summoning up first aid he had learned in a high school class, tried to make the youngster comfortable. He ducked through a side door to his garage, retrieved a set of folded beach towels lying on the clothes dryer, and ran back out to cover the boy. Even as he was preparing to check the unconscious child's head for bleeding, the boy's parents pushed their way through the crowd of men, women, and children who had been summoned to the scene by the sound of screeching brakes. As Bobby's mother and father knelt to their son, the sounds of an approaching helicopter swept over the street.

The crowd lined itself up against the garage door and the side of the house. Gingerly, the helicopter, the "COIT HILL TRAUMA CENTER" insignia painted on its belly growing larger and sharper, descended into the wide street. Two paramedics jumped out and ran to the fallen youngster.

"Okay, son, you've done fine," one said quietly to the teenager, who was shaking violently. "Let us take over." The other man took the child's mother—who was now sitting next to her son, stroking his head—by the shoulders and gently helped her up. "It'd be better if you move too, lady." The boy's father, who had been crouching next to her, stood, nodded, and led her a few feet away.

As the teenager and the parents backed away, one of the paramedics quickly opened the trauma box he had brought with him and took out a blood-pressure cuff. "Get a backboard," he told his partner as he adjusted the cuff on the boy's thin arm and began to pump on the small black rubber bulb.

The other man ran back to the craft and brought the backboard and a collar for the boy's neck. Working together, the two men fitted the collar then lifted the boy carefully and placed him on the hard stretcher. "Okay," one of the paramedics said, "let's get an IV going."

Oblivious to the sounds of the mother crying in the background, the paramedics pushed a needle into the crook of the boy's arm, then connected it to a plastic bag filled with a clear liquid. With carefully synchronized movements, they lifted the stretcher and carried the boy to the helicopter.

The woman grabbed the paramedic's arm. "Couldn't we call an ambulance? I don't know . . . that other Coit Hill helicopter . . ."

"Ma'am, the other copter crash was a fluke. I've flown out of smaller areas in Nam. There's no danger, ma'am."

The woman would not let go of his arm. The paramedic took hold of her hand and pried it loose. "We're wasting time, ma'am. He'll be fine, believe me. We'll get him there in plenty of time."

"Let them go, Liz," her husband said softly. "The man's right."

Accompanied by the whine and roar of straining engines, the helicopter shot into the air, made a sharp right turn over the rooftops, and disappeared.

Julie, curled into a chair in Allan's living room, put down her book and watched Allan pace around the living room.

"Allan, sit down and relax. You're not going to make the time go faster by marching around here all evening and all night."

"I can't Julie. Darnit, why couldn't Younger get the story into tonight's edition of the Sunday paper? It would all be over by now."

"He explained it to you a dozen times. He didn't get back from L.A. until eleven this morning. There was no way he could make the deadline. It'll be in the morning paper."

"But . . ."

"That's soon enough, babe." Julie walked to the kitchen and came back with the entertainment section of the *Telegraph*. "Come on," she said. "Let's get a bite to eat and see a movie."

Everett Huntington watched for a second as Cluny and another nurse, caring for the boy brought in by the helicopter, moved rapidly through the resuscitation routines he had drilled them on. Satisfied, he picked up one of the five telephones he had ordered installed in strategic places around the emergency room. The anesthesiologist whose number he had dialed was at home.

"I've timed the run," he told Huntington. "I'll be there in twelve minutes."

Huntington clenched his fist and shook it in self-tribute, then ran his finger down the on-call list until he came to the name of a surgeon who had some experience with children and who lived less than twenty minutes away. The physician was walking in after a day in which he had performed minor surgical procedures in a free clinic, but said he would be at Coit Hill hard on the anesthesiologist's heels.

For once, Huntington said to himself with a great deal of satisfaction, something is going to go right around here.

The phone rang as he was studying the second round of lab tests he had ordered. He let it ring as he concentrated on the figures, assuring himself that they backed up his initial diagnosis that the youngster was losing blood internally and that surgery was needed to stop the hemorrhaging. Finally he took the phone off the hook. It was Sherman Harper.

"Who have you got on call tonight, Everett?" Harper asked.

"Herbert for anesthesiology and Dysan for surgery. They are—"

"Tremendous! Get them in for me, will you?"

"They're—"

"Listen, don't interrupt. I've got a lady on whom we were going to do a triple bypass Monday. She's showing signs of an infarction and I want to go in before the damage spreads."

"Sherman, hold on, will you? I've already got Herbert and Dysan coming in. We've got a pediatric trauma case in. Kid on a bike got hit by a car."

"Well, call the backup team. It's a good thing you have Herbert, the man's terrific with anesthesia in cardiac cases. I use him all the time."

"Sherman, I need to get that kid in the O.R. within the hour."

"Then stop wasting our time and get on the phone and get the backup anesthesiologist and surgeon in. I'm taking Herbert and Dysan."

"You can't do that, Sherman!"

"What do you mean I can't do that? I've got a sixty-two-year-old lady who needs help stat. I already have the pump team coming in. The kid can hold out a little longer until you get someone else in." The phone went dead as Harper hung up.

Without hesitating, Huntington began dialing the next number on the list. When, within a span of seven minutes, he had talked to four surgeons and three anesthesiologists and had not been able to recruit another team, Huntington dialed a number that was not part of the neatly typed list. The boy, he estimated, had another forty minutes of life left. The call he was making would probably cost him, but he was not about to allow a child to die for the sake of Anthony's pride.

"Allan," Julie said in mock exasperation as she watched him twirl his spoon again and again around the small espresso cup. "Would you mind joining me for a few minutes this evening?"

He looked up at her, his eyes reflecting worry. "Do you think I did the right thing?"

"In giving Younger the study?"

Allan nodded.

Julie put down the cup she had lifted to her lips. "Do you want to know the truth?"

He nodded again.

"I don't know. You had to do it. But I don't know if it was the right thing to do in terms of what has happened to you."

"What's happened to me hardly matters. It couldn't get worse, anyway. I mean, was it the right thing to do in terms of changing things?"

"That we won't know until we see what the reaction is, from

the public, the politicians, and, for that matter, from the hospitals. Drink up, kid, or we'll be late for the show."

Huntington, his eyes fixed on the clock, grew increasingly impatient as the voice coming at him through the telephone droned on.

"Fedder," he finally interrupted, "I know all about the county transfer requirements. Yes, the child is highly unstable. But I can't get anyone in here to operate. That boy is going to bleed out on us unless we go in."

"And I'm telling you that I can't authorize the transfer. Everett, you don't know what it's been like around here since all the shit with Kirk broke. If we accept that transfer and the kid dies, even if he dies in the ambulance on the way over here, that death would be our responsibility. We just can't handle one more thing going wrong. Any other time, I'd say fuck it, send him over. But not now, Everett. I'm sorry."

"Wait!" Huntington yelled. "Don't hang up."

"Everett . . ."

"No. Hold on a sec. Let me think."

"Everett, I've got work to do."

Huntington stopped to take a deep breath. "David, listen. Can you send a trauma team over here to operate on him?"

"Are you out of your skull, Everett? In the first place that would leave us uncovered here. . . ."

"You've got a backup team. They'd be in almost before you were out the door."

"Everett. None of us has O.R. privileges over there. And I for one don't want to spend the rest of my life teaching at the University of Acapulco."

Huntington glanced at the clock. Fifteen minutes had gone by. He had already given the boy four pints of blood. He had a chest tube in. But his vital signs and the reports from the lab showed he was losing ground. If they were lucky, he had twenty-five minutes to live.

"You don't need privileges. Look, we're set up now to do operations within our emergency room for cases that can't wait to go up to the regular O.R. All I need to do is to get some additional equipment down here. A laparotomy set, some vascular instruments. I'm the director of the E.R. so I'll take full responsibility for what needs to be done. You won't have to answer to anyone."

There was silence on the other side.

"Fedder, a little boy is dying. . . ."

Fedder squeezed his eyes shut, put his free hand under the pit of the arm with which he was holding the phone, and leaned forward, the picture of a man hit by a sudden attack of stomach cramps. "You fucker, if you are messing with me . . ."

"I'm not lying to you, Dave."

"Okay," Fedder whispered. "I've got Jergens here on anesthesiology. . . ."

Huntington was ecstatic. "Terrific, his specialty is pediatric anesthesiology."

"And a woman intern who's so gaga over Kirk she's kicking over a psychiatric residency at Menninger to stay here for trauma training. If I can get them to agree, if I can get a backup team to come in, and if there is an ambulance around . . ."

"Never mind the ambulance," Huntington said, elated even more by the delicious idea that had just struck him. "I'll send Anthony's new helicopter to pick you up."

"Like hell you will. I'd rather walk."

"Don't be an asshole, David. I know the pilot. This one knows what he's doing."

"I'm glad somebody around there does," Fedder grumbled, and hung up.

Huntington was standing at the boy's side when he heard the helicopter returning from the University. The boy's blood pressure, which he had coaxed up earlier to 90/70 with additional fluids, had slipped to 60/40. The child's skin felt cool, clammy to the touch. His abdomen, filling with blood, was swelling relentlessly.

"Well, you fuck up, you leave the hallowed halls of academia, and these are your just rewards," a voice boomed behind him. It was Fedder, and behind him were another man and a young woman. Huntington hugged Fedder and planted a wet kiss on his cheek.

"Okay, okay, never mind the sissy stuff," Fedder said, freeing himself from Huntington's grasp and making a show of wiping his face. "That our patient?"

"That's him," Huntington said, looking around for someone to help them transfer the child on to the operating table. He beckoned to Cluny, but she only threw him an icy stare. A vocational nurse who had wandered into the emergency room caught Huntington's motion and came over to volunteer.

"I'll fill you in while we scrub," Huntington said. But even though he began to recite all the necessary facts and figures, a part of his mind was away from the scene, wrestling with the look of censure he had caught in Cluny's eyes.

Huntington had all but forgotten Cluny's hateful glare, the argument he had had with Harper, the difficulty he had had persuading Fedder to shuttle over to Coit Hill when, some two hours later, he and his colleagues were gathered around the boy's bedside.

"He looks good, I guess," Fedder said, pride evident in his voice.

"Terrific!" Huntington answered. "The three of you did a hell of a job in there."

"We still have a problem, you know," Fedder said. "The kid is really officially our patient now. I'd like to take him back to the University with us."

Huntington contemplated the sleeping boy, taken by the relaxed expression on his face. "We could transfer him now, but I'm not sure it's really necessary," he answered.

"And if there are complications?"

"There won't be. You did your job in there and his signs have been strong and stable for a good half hour without any extraordinary support from us. There won't be any surprises."

"Still . . ."

"If you're worried about a consult, I've got that covered. Harper's case should be about done, so when Dysan comes out of surgery I'll ask him to take on the boy. He'll do a fine job with him."

They walked away from the bed, Fedder and Huntington

trailing behind Maggie and the University anesthesiologist. Fedder signaled Huntington to slow down.

"Everett, not to change the subject, but are you happy here?"

"The money is good," Huntington answered evasively. "And there are challenges."

"Like what? Seeing if your buddies will rush over from another hospital to take care of a patient your hospital can't handle?"

"That's not fair, Dave," Huntington shot back, then paused. "Oh, hell, I guess it is."

"So I repeat the question. You happy?"

"No, I guess not. All the trappings are here. But . . . well, no, I guess I'm really not."

"So what are you going to do?"

"I don't know," Huntington said, knowing full well he was lying to his friend. A course of action had sprung up in his mind while he had been waiting for the helicopter to get back from the University. It was a plan that had jelled as he had watched Fedder operate. The only question that remained was whether he had the guts to carry it out.

After they made love, quietly and leisurely, Julie quickly fell asleep. Allan remained wide awake. At least a dozen times during the long night he rose to pace the apartment, to look in the refrigerator for something to eat, to read a few pages of a medical journal, to look out at the deserted street. Several times he had to fight the temptation to shake Julie out of her sleep and ask her to sit down for some coffee and some conversation. He considered, but dismissed, the possibility of going to the *Telegraph* building and begging a copy of the morning edition from one of the people who would be loading the bundles of newspapers onto the delivery trucks.

At six fifteen he could no longer contain himself. He threw on a sweatshirt and jeans and ran down to the corner. The store was dark. Stacked near the door were two bundles of newspapers. He paced up and down but Kee Park, the old Korean who owned the store, did not appear. Allan decided on a quick ten-minute jog and ran off. When he returned, the store was still dark and Kee was nowhere in sight. Allan looked up one street, down another. Then, telling himself that he would pay Park later in the morning, he reached down and tugged a paper out of the top bundle.

Julie, fast asleep, was on her back, one arm and one leg sprawled into the area of the bed where he should have been. For a moment he hesitated. But his eagerness to share what he had strained to read in the breaking dawn as he walked home pushed aside the feeling of consideration. He sat down on the edge of the bed, leaned over, and kissed her on the lips. She smiled, stirred, and, without opening her eyes, rolled away toward her side of the bed. He leaned over and kissed her again, just below her ear. She squirmed, purred, but seemed to settle deeper into the bed. Frustrated, Allan smacked her rear end with the folded paper. "Julie, wake up! I've got the paper."

With a jerk she twisted back toward him and propped herself up on her elbows. She opened, then closed, then opened her eyes again.

"I got the *Telegraph*," he repeated.

"The what?" She shook her head, tried to focus on Allan. "Oh. What's it say?"

"It's good stuff, want to hear?"

She pushed herself higher on the bed and the cover slipped off her body. Instinctively, Allan's gaze dropped to her breasts.

"Forget it," she said, now fully awake and laughing. "Not after being so rudely awakened. Go make some coffee, I'll be there in a minute."

Allan, bubbling with excitement, filled the percolator basket with coffee, poured water into the pot, and plugged it in. He heard the toilet flush, then Julie shuffling toward the kitchen.

"What has the man written?"

"Listen:

Almost half of all critically injured patients taken to San Francisco County hospital emergency rooms may be dying because those hospitals cannot provide the care needed to save the patients' lives, the *Telegraph* has learned.

According to a study obtained by the *Telegraph*, of 100

patients who died in community hospitals over a thirteen-month period spanning the last two years, 45 died because:

- A number of emergency rooms are staffed by physicians who are not emergency-care specialists. In many cases, physicians on duty in these emergency rooms were not able to diagnose in time the injuries afflicting the patients.
- Even when qualified emergency-room doctors diagnosed injuries correctly, they had difficulty reaching surgeons and specialists who were needed to provide definitive care for the patients. The problem has been particularly acute at night.

The study was conducted by Dr. Allan Kirk, a University of California trauma surgeon, and Julie McDonough, a statistics specialist with the San Francisco County Medical Examiner.

Kirk is on leave from the University while officials investigate his use of an artificial blood compound in a trauma patient. Kirk is also facing censure as a result of his outspoken criticism of community hospital treatment of critically injured patients.

Kirk's data and his interpretation of care given the deceased patients in his study, however, were independently confirmed by two trauma experts contacted by the *Telegraph*.

'The data is almost irrefutable,' Dr. Harold Sykes, a professor of surgery at the University of Southern California Medical School told the *Telegraph*. 'Not every one of the patients he found could have been saved. But many who died did so because critical surgery was not performed or not performed in time.'

A second surgeon, who agreed to review Kirk's findings but who declined to be identified, also concurred that up to half of the deaths in the sample could have been prevented with better and faster medical care."

Allan stopped.
"That's it?" Julie asked.

"No, it goes on," he said, his voice crackling with excitement, his eyes sparkling. "We're going to have the bastards running for their lives. There isn't a trauma team in the world that's going to be skilled enough to save their asses." With a shout of joy, he threw the newspaper high in the air. Julie came over, sat on his lap, and bent down to give him a long kiss.

He was grinning from ear to ear. "You know what I'm going to love? Walking into that conference tomorrow."

Julie pulled back a bit so she could see him better. "What conference?"

"Hell, I forgot to tell you. I got a call while you were out Friday. There is going to be a second settlement conference at the University on the biker suit. I'm going to love to see just how those bastards react to this. Ha!"

"Not too well, I imagine," she said. "But the hell with tomorrow. Let's celebrate. Let's drive down to Carmel and have a dinner and—"

The clamoring of the phone interrupted her and they both turned to look at it.

"At seven-fifteen on a Sunday morning?" Julie asked.

He lifted her off his lap and picked up the receiver. He turned slowly to her as he listened. "KIT-TV," he mouthed silently.

Al Anthony was slumped in his easy chair. His chin was deep in his throat. His arms were folded across his chest. When he heard the doorbell, he pushed himself to his feet and walked backward to the front door of his apartment, never taking his eyes off the screen. He turned the doorknob, glanced back quickly to make sure it was Cummings he was allowing entrance, and headed back to his chair.

"The cocksucker has been going on like that on every news program I turn to," Anthony said, pointing to Allan's image on the television.

"How are you, Harrison? Have a nice Sunday, Harrison? Why, yes, thank you, Al. Very nice."

"Fuck you, Harrison. Where the hell have you been? I've been trying to call you since early this morning."

"Yes, Al, I'd love a beer. Where have I been? Out. There are limitations, you know, even to being at your beck and call."

"Not right now, there aren't. The beer is in the refrigerator, help yourself. Have you heard what's going on?"

"The Kirk study?" Cummings called out as he went to the kitchen. "My gosh, what a mess, Anthony. How can you live with a sink full of dishes like this? Yes, I heard snatches about it on one of the all-news radio stations." He walked back into the living room and pulled a wooden rocker over next to Anthony's easy chair.

"Listen to this." Anthony rose and pushed buttons on the video recording device beneath his television. "I recorded this half an hour ago on the early-evening news on Channel Seven. They gave the bastard almost ten minutes of airtime. I'll skip all the crap that was in the paper and get to the really good parts."

Static and snow covered the screen; then Allan and a young woman, a microphone in her hand, materialized on the screen. Like characters in a silent movie, Allan and the woman exchanged exaggerated mouth and hand movements. When a graph flashed on the screen, Anthony slowed down the tape.

". . . but what is interesting is not just how many people are dying, Clare," Allan was saying. "What is even more important is who is dying and where they are dying. The chart clearly shows us that trauma is a devastating event because it is one of the leading killers of young people, not just in San Francisco, but in the country generally. In our study, fifty-two percent of the people who died needlessly were between the ages of sixteen and thirty-six. And that's not all. Another thirty percent of our sample were men and women between the ages of thirty-seven and fifty-seven. So if you look at it carefully, you find that eight out of ten people who die needlessly are people who are probably working, supporting families, contributing to society. Trauma kills people who are either in the most productive years of their lives or about to enter them."

"Interesting. But you said that what was important too was where people were dying. Are you referring to Coit Hill?"

"Listen to this shit, Harrison," Anthony interjected.

On the television, Allan smiled at the interviewer. "No, not at all. I think that people have gotten the impression that only Coit Hill has a problem handling trauma. But almost every hospital has difficulties."

"Is it mostly the smaller hospitals, then?"

"No, that's precisely the point. In our sample, more than half of the unnecessary deaths took place in the large hospitals, those that have two hundred and fifty beds or more, the hospitals that are supposed to have all of the world's best facilities."

"So you really can't trust any hospital in San Francisco?"

"And that cunt is playing right into his hands, can you believe it?" Anthony commented.

Allan shook his head. "You may be able to trust them to take your gallbladder out. But not for trauma. No."

Anthony stood up and turned the machine off. "Let's take a look at the six o'clock news," he said. "I bet he's on there as well."

The program had already started. Allan and the newscaster, an Asian man, were deep into their interview.

". . . and so the answer is what, Dr. Kirk?"

"The answer is simple. The Board of Supervisors must ask all hospitals in San Francisco interested in becoming a trauma center to submit full applications detailing how they would design, fund, and run such a center. The applications should then be evaluated by a group of outside experts and they should recommend one hospital to receive the designation. The hospital that would get the designation would commit itself to hiring surgeons and anesthesiologists who would dedicate themselves only to trauma patients and who would be in-house when the patients arrive. The hospital would also have to promise, in effect, always to keep an operating room free for potential victims and to have sufficient support services to get the patients through the crucial post-op period."

"That sounds simple, all right. But if it is, why hasn't it been done?"

"Because hospitals don't want to take the chance that they won't get the designation, so they oppose the concept. In extreme cases like Coit Hill's, they set up ex-officio trauma centers in the hope of executing an end run around any potential designation competition."

"But isn't that what you tried to do at the University?" The newscaster looked smug, proud of the way he had sprung his trap.

"Answer that, you dumb shit!" Anthony yelled at the television.

"That is true," Allan said, struggling to maintain his composure. "The only excuse we have is that in light of the vacuum in the county, we organized a trauma team because we at least know that we can gather a group of professionals that is truly dedicated to trauma care. And that is more than I can say for the other hospitals."

Anthony stood. "I can't take this crap anymore."

"Keep it on, Al," Cummings said. "Let's hear him out."

". . . My feeling is," Allan continued, "that insofar as trauma care is concerned, we are in a state of anarchy and that people will continue to die unless the public demands that one official center is named."

"Demands? How?"

"By showing that it won't tolerate the situation. The citizens of this city should write their supervisors, meet with hospital boards, hit the hospitals in the pocketbook."

"That sounds very close to calling for a boycott, Dr. Kirk."

Anthony's mouth dropped open. He turned to Cummings. "The man is a bigger maniac than even I thought, Harrison."

"Al, shut up!" Cummings rose to turn up the volume on the set.

"Well, I don't know if that is really possible," Allan said. "But hospitals are sensitive to economic pressures since most of them operate on the tightest budgets imaginable. It's not hard to imagine that the public could take some of their hospital business, like elective surgeries or diagnostic tests, to other facilities nearby, say in Marin. I think the hospitals would get the message rather quickly."

The newscaster shook his head, working hard to show his amazement. "That is certainly a novel approach, Dr. Kirk. But where is all this going to leave you with the medical community? You are already in hot water and now you are asking for a public revolt against them."

"At this point I haven't got very much to lose. And I simply don't care."

"I'll give you plenty to care about, you asshole," Anthony fumed.

Cummings waved to him to keep quiet.

". . . I have made a decision to put my career on hold. . . ."

"In the ash can, you mean, you jerk."

Cummings shushed him.

"This one issue," Allan was saying, "is more important to me than anything else. We all need to make the hard decisions now. If we blow it, if we allow hospital administrators like Al Anthony to give us half-baked, showcase trauma plans that are just empty shells, we will go on needlessly losing lives. I am willing to take my chances with my future and invest my energy on this one project. Even if the project fails, I at least will know in my heart that I have done everything humanly possible."

Anthony leaped out of his chair and punched the power button on the television set. "That's about as much of that crap as I can take."

He walked to the wet bar tucked away in a corner of his apartment and poured himself a glass of bourbon and water. He held the liquor bottle up to Cummings. "This or another beer?"

"The bourbon."

He poured Cummings a generous portion. He handed it to the lawyer, then went to the picture window to open the drapes, exposing, from the fifteenth-floor apartment in his Embarcadero condominium, the lights of the city. For two or three minutes he stared out at San Francisco.

"The man is incredible," he said to Cummings without turning around. "You almost have to admire him. We get him booted out of the University, we get his research funding cut off, we put Bumqua on his tail, and he goes on like nothing is happening."

Anthony came back to his easy chair and sat down. Cummings, studying the administrator's face, could see the moment of calm was over. "Who the hell does this guy think he is?" Anthony asked. "Doing a study like that on his own, releasing it without even giving the hospital council a chance to react to it?" He stood up, walked back to the window, walked back to face Cummings. "And who the hell is this guy Younger to print this kind of shit? No review of the data by the editorial board of a medical journal. Nothing. But they just slap it out there on the front page, like it was God's own truth!"

"Well, you know the media," Cummings answered calmly. "Always looking for an excuse to tear things down."

"Whores, but never mind them. What can we do about Kirk?" Anthony stopped. "Shit, and on top of this we have the settlement conference with the University people tomorrow."

"That conference is the least of your worries. I don't think they give a rat's ass about Kirk anymore or his studies. So this won't affect our discussions there. But as to what you and I can do about Kirk, you won't like my answer, but at this point I don't think very much. Al, you've shot your load."

"There's always something that can be done. Get some experts to look at his data and prove he's wrong. A libel suit, a—"

"No one's been libeled, Al. And as far as getting 'experts' to look at his data to prove he's wrong, do you think he is?"

"That's beside the point."

"No, it's not really. Do you think he's wrong?"

"Well, I . . ."

"All right, then don't talk about taking that route. It would only backfire on you anyway."

Cummings got up and poured himself more bourbon, then took a sip. "Of course, the daring and brilliant thing to do would be to go public and say that Kirk is right." Cummings gave Anthony a broad grin.

"You're loony."

"No, listen to me. How much more can you hurt Kirk? Not much. You just ticked off everything we've already done. And I think you know that his data on the deaths is pretty unassailable. So why not approach this from the positive side, which is that Kirk has given you a hell of an opportunity."

"Which is exactly what?"

"Kirk has the public's attention now. He has pointed out dramatically that what San Francisco needs is a single trauma center. That's what you want too. He has done a lot of your work for you."

"But he's talking about a competition for the designation.

Any one of half a dozen hospitals, including the University, would go for it."

"Just follow along for a moment. All right, Kirk has roused the public, has made a great case for an individual trauma center. At the same time, he is out there all by his lonesome. No support from the hospital council. No support from the medical community, which doesn't like free-lancers like him, no support anymore even from his own institution."

"So?"

"So why don't *we* offer him support. Tell him we've been wrong. Convince him that you were well meaning in your earlier objections, but now that you've seen his study, that you have seen the light. Offer him two hundred thou a year to come on board, to write the proposal that would win the designation, to actually set up the center. No strings attached. Same deal you gave Harper and Huntington. To sweeten the pot offer him private funding for his blood research."

"Cummings, your coke habit is starting to eat your brain. Some tough weekend you must have had."

"Think about it. Without you at this point, all he's got is the possible glory of having pushed San Francisco into having a trauma center. After that, what? Nothing. He's a shattered man, someone whose career is in a shambles and, crusading fervor or no, he has to realize that. What we'll be offering him is a chance to join hands with the county's most powerful hospital administrator not just to build his dream, but to save his ass as well."

"Can I ask you something? Suppose he doesn't go along with us?"

"Then play hardball."

"We've already done that."

"But maybe not hard enough."

Anthony contemplated his lawyer. "You talking about bumping him off?"

Cummings laughed. "Don't be ridiculous. But maybe we should find out who this Julie McDonough is and what she means to him. Somebody in that relationship has to have some smarts."

15

Anger built up in Anthony again as he listened to the Monday morning radio news on his way in to work. And, as he marched into Coit Hill, the snatches of interviews with Allan, interviews with other hospital administrators making hysterical denials of culpability, not to mention a two-minute editorial by the manager of the station demanding a response to Allan's study, still hammered at him. But, determined as he was to get to his desk and start his counteroffensive, he found himself slowed by the slightly bemused expression his executive secretary liked to put on when she was privy to something he did not yet know. He glanced at the door to his office and saw that it was open. That meant she had shown someone in to await his arrival. Moving quietly, he took care to change his path so that he could not be seen from inside his office as he approached the secretary's desk.

"Who?" he whispered when he was close to her.

"Cluny."

He rolled his eyes upward in exasperation, simultaneously feeling his chest tighten slightly in foreboding.

"Well! Miss Cluny, what a pleasure!" he said with forced enthusiasm. "What can I do for you so early in the day?"

Cluny, as usual, was perched on the edge of the chair, her hands clasped on her lap. Her face, though, was haggard. Anthony remembered she was on night duty. That meant she had made an extra effort to stay up after her shift in order to be in his office first thing in the morning. The sense that he was about to receive news of an impending—or already occurred—disaster grew stronger.

Cluny straightened out a bit. "I do not enjoy having to come to you like this, Mr. Anthony," she opened. "But I feel I have no choice. No one else seems to care very much about what goes on in this institution."

Anthony by now had put down his attaché case, had taken off and hung up his jacket, and had taken his seat behind his desk. "As I have indicated before, Miss Cluny, I appreciate your conscientiousness." He gave her an expansive smile.

"Last night a young boy who had been struck by an automobile was brought into the emergency room by our helicopter rescue squad. Dr. Huntington called upon Doctors Herbert and Dysan, but unfortunately about the same time Dr. Harper had to take a case into the operating room. Since Dr. Herbert is expert in anesthesia involving cardiac patients, Dr. Harper requested his services. He also requested that Dr. Dysan assist him."

Anthony smiled and nodded for her to go on.

She took a deep breath, as if to underscore that she was being forced to do something thoroughly distasteful to her. "Dr. Huntington made one or two calls to find a backup team. But, rather than go on trying, Dr. Huntington called the University . . ."

". . . and had the boy transferred," Anthony finished for her, relieved that her complaint would probably only be that Huntington had not complied with all the complicated transfer rules and regulations.

Disgust was written all over Cluny's face, as if she were about to drop soiled underwear on his desk.

"No, Mr. Anthony, he did not. The University refused the transfer. Instead, at Dr. Huntington's insistence, they sent a surgical team over here to operate on the boy."

There was silence. "I'm sorry," Anthony said, puzzled, convinced he had misunderstood. "Did you say that a surgical team from the University came over here to operate on one of our patients?"

"Well, technically he wasn't our patient yet," said Cluny, ever the stickler for form and propriety. "As you well know, emergency-room patients do not become ours until someone formally admits them. But, yes, that is exactly what I said. A team from the University operated on the boy here."

"I see," Anthony said, though in truth he did not. To stall for time, he buzzed his secretary and asked for his morning coffee, all the while wildly trying to calculate what this new turn meant. Were Huntington and Kirk allied somehow? Was this part of a new plot to embarrass him and Coit Hill?

"I'm sorry," he said, addressing Cluny again. "Would you like some coffee?"

"Please," she said with an air that clearly conveyed her hurt in not having been asked immediately. Anthony, glad to have a few more seconds to think, buzzed his secretary again and asked her to bring a second cup in.

"Did the University people take the boy with them afterward?"

The secretary came in with the coffees, then gracefully retired.

"No. No, they did not. When Dr. Dysan was finished assisting Dr. Harper with his cardiac case, Dr. Huntington asked Dr. Dysan to admit the boy. There was a bit of a discussion, but Dr. Dysan did accede to Dr. Huntington's request. The boy is in our ICU. I checked on him before I came in. His condition is satisfactory. Nevertheless . . ."

She stopped as Anthony lunged for his telephone and buzzed his secretary. When she answered he asked her to hold on. "Thank you, Miss Cluny," he said, standing up to signal that the meeting had come to an end. "I appreciate your bringing this to my attention."

"I didn't think there was anything else to do," she replied, her chin high and her lips taut. "It was clearly my duty."

An hour later, an exhausted Everett Huntington was sitting in the chair Cluny had vacated. Anthony picked up a two-inch-thick book and threw it on Huntington's lap. Thinking about the incident later, Huntington was almost convinced that Anthony had tried to throw it so that one edge would land squarely against his groin.

"If you'll open that," Anthony said, fury curling around every word, "you'll see that the text is divided into two sections. The first part is a copy of this hospital's bylaws. The second is a copy of the Northern California Hospital Council's rules, regulations, and standards of ethics. Take your time, Dr. Huntington, while you try to find, in either section, the paragraph that makes an allowance for surgeons who do not have privileges at an institution to dance in and operate on a patient there."

Huntington slowly picked up the book and put it back on Anthony's desk.

"Al, let's not play games."

"Good idea, Everett, good idea." Anthony got up and walked toward Huntington. Anthony eased himself down against one edge of the desk, folded his arms across his chest, then leaned forward.

"If we are not playing games here," he continued, "then can you explain to me just exactly what it was you were doing last night, inviting University people to come over here and operate on that boy?" Anthony straightened up. "Go ahead and take your time."

"I wasn't playing any kind of game. I needed surgical help for the boy. I couldn't get it from the people on our on-call list, so I did what I thought was best to save his life."

"What you thought was best to save his life." The statement came out flat, yet dripping in sarcasm. "And that included bringing in physicians without privileges."

"Technically, they didn't need privileges because they didn't operate in one of our surgical suites. They operated in the emergency operating room on an accident victim who had not yet been admitted to the hospital. I felt that under those circumstances I could bring them in as consultants to me."

Anthony blinked as he processed the information. "That's

beside the point," he snarled when he understood what Huntington was telling him. "Just how do you think we'll look when it gets out that we had to have University people in here to take care of one of our emergency-room cases!"

"That we care more about the lives of the people that depend on us than about our pride?"

"You idiot! Don't you think you could have waited an hour for Harper to get through with his case?"

Huntington was tired, but not too tired to realize that at the end of the conversation Anthony would probably fire him. And having decided that his future at Coit Hill could be measured in terms of minutes, he decided to make the best of his situation. "In my estimation," he finally answered, "there wasn't even enough time to wait for the University team to take an ambulance over." He looked directly at Anthony. "Which is why I even sent your helicopter to get them."

Anthony opened his mouth, but no sound emerged. He closed it again. Anthony went back to his leather chair. He shuffled through the papers his secretary had put in his in-basket, picked out a folder, and started to look through its contents. "You're finished at this hospital, Huntington," he said in a low voice. "You're through. Don't let me see your face here again."

Huntington pushed himself out of the chair and left the office. He took an elevator to the hospital's basement and, with the help of a janitor, found about half a dozen empty boxes and took them to his office. He cleaned out his files, discarding correspondence and records he did not need, packing journals, medical books, and notes he had accumulated for articles he might someday write. The janitor stacked the boxes on a dolly and, taking Huntington's car keys from the doctor, backed out of the office, pulling the load after him.

When the man had cleared the threshold, Huntington closed and locked the office door. He took a small chain holding two thin keys out of a compartment in his wallet and, kneeling, used one of the keys to unlock a black two-drawer file cabinet standing between his desk and the wall. He had ordered the cabinet so he could store sensitive and important material. But the metallic rattling of the top drawer as he pulled it open bore testimony to the fact that during his few months at Coit Hill he had had occasion to put only one file in there. He took out the four folders that made up the file and put them in the briefcase his wife had given him as a present when he took the job at Coit Hill. He folded the thin leather strap over the top of the briefcase, pressed the snap shut, then locked it with the second small key on his chain. That done, he typed out a memo explaining his departure to his staff and posted it on the bulletin board behind the emergency-room reception counter. He looked around, then walked out.

Anthony, getting off the elevator on his way to the second settlement conference with the University people, spotted Cummings walking ahead of him.

"Harrison!"

The lawyer stopped and turned around. Anthony caught up to him and pulled him to the side of the hall.

"Do you think we can get this postponed?" Anthony whispered. "There's just too much happening at once for me to deal with." Talking quickly, Anthony filled Cummings in on the events involving the University trauma team and Huntington. "And to boot," he went on, "I got a call from two of the supervisors demanding that I convene an immediate meeting of the Joint Committee for Emergency Services to deal with the Kirk study."

"And did you?"

"What the hell else could I do? I set it for tomorrow night. What a fuckin' mess!"

Together they resumed walking to the conference room, but Anthony stopped. "We've got to talk to Kirk, see if we can sell him on your idea."

Cummings studied his shoes, then looked up at Anthony. "I already did."

"You what? When?"

"I called him at seven this morning and asked him to meet me for breakfast or something. Actually, he surprised me and agreed to hear what I had to say."

"Well? What did he say to the proposal about coming to work at Coit?"

"You mean after he stopped laughing? He turned me down flat. I tried reasoning with him, tried to point out that an alliance with you would make him the most powerful trauma physician in the county, that he could have everything he wanted. But he wouldn't bite. Wasn't even tempted to nibble."

They stopped talking as Phil Dorr, University hospital administrator Jack White, and attorneys Joyce Cole and Randolph Astor swept by.

"We'd better go in," Cummings said. "But I don't think it would be a bad idea to consider our alternative plan. In fact, I've already made the necessary arrangements. I just have to make a phone call to put them into effect."

"Our alternative plan?"

"To talk to Ms. McDonough," Cummings said as they walked briskly into the conference room and shook hands with the University people.

There was no easy chatter; there were neither doughnuts nor the ingredients for coffee.

"Does anyone know if Dr. Kirk remembers this meeting?" Joyce Cole asked.

"I had my office call him and—" Dorr began, but stopped as Allan strolled in. Though the others merely nodded toward him or mumbled hellos, Dorr stood to welcome Allan with a handshake. "Right on time," Dorr said. "Let's get started."

"If you don't mind, let's wait a minute," Allan answered. "A couple of people came with me, but they had to make a pit stop." He smiled warmly at the group, as if they had gathered for a friendly poker game.

A minute later an elderly gentleman, tall, thin, somewhat stooped, ambled in. He had a gentle, grandfatherly air about him. Dorr, who had taken his seat again after greeting Allan, almost leaped out of his chair. "Walter Creighton!" he said with unrestrained enthusiasm. "I haven't seen you for a good four or five years!"

Dorr turned to the rest of the group. "For those of you who

don't know," and the blank stares on all their faces told him they indeed had no idea who the man was, "Dr. Creighton was—sorry, is—one of the nation's most eminent pathologists." Dorr's voice lost some of its thrill and volume when the implications of Creighton's potential role in the discussion began to dawn on him. "He was head of Stanford's pathology department," he finished in much more subdued fashion, "until his retirement seven years ago."

Creighton's appearance had unsettled only Dorr. But when Allan's second companion entered, the effect on the entire group would have been no less had Allan stood at the doorway and tossed a live grenade on the conference table. Roger Steinhardt's round face—along with the round wire glasses that framed dark, flashing eyes; the abundant mustache, the salt-and-pepper hair arranged in a perm cut—was familiar to them all. White, Dorr, and Anthony knew the face from its frequent appearance over the last fifteen years on the Bay area's front pages and television programs. On several occasions, Joyce Cole had faced Steinhardt in court, and she had lost the majority of her legal confrontations with him.

Allan took command having noted the consternation and confusion Creighton and Steinhardt's appearance had caused. "If you are expecting some kind of an opening statement from me, you'll be disappointed. I just have one thing to say and that is that I will not be a party to the settlement that was discussed here when we last met. Unless we can work out something more satisfactory today, I am prepared to go to court on the matter."

Dorr took great pains to look and sound friendly. "Allan . . ."

"Phil, save your breath. You're not going to sacrifice my life and my career for the sake of your University. I'm going to fight this, and I don't give a damn what you think about it."

"Surely, Dr. Kirk," Cole interjected, "even as unhappy as you are, you must realize how tenuous your legal situation is. What is the point of making matters even more difficult?"

"Surely *you* must realize that my client's position is tenuous only as long as he is not afforded a defense," Steinhardt said before Allan had a chance to reply.

"Have you looked at the records, Roger? Have you had time to study this case?"

"I won't even consider that a serious question, Joyce."

"I think, then," she continued, "that we can pretty much agree on the basic issues, can't we?"

"Which are?"

"That your client, Dr. Kirk, performed an unauthorized experimental procedure on the young man in question who would otherwise have had a reasonable chance of surviving. And second, that he failed even to obtain the family's consent to carry out that procedure—assuming, of course, that the family could validly have consented to the use of the artificial blood."

"I see. Let's take that last assertion first, shall we? For my information, please tell me why you think that Dr. Kirk did not have permission to carry out his allegedly experimental procedure?"

"Oh, come on, Roger! Do you see anywhere in that file the form used by every reputable researcher when he or she is using an experimental drug or procedure which is approved for human beings?"

"No, I don't, but that does not mean that my client did not have permission to use his artificial blood formula."

"Mr. Steinhardt, there is simply no way that is possible," Anthony interrupted. "Dr. Kirk did nothing to obtain that family's acquiescence to his little scheme."

"That I grant you, Mr. Anthony," Steinhardt said, while reaching into his attaché case and pulling out a three-page document.

Anthony instantly recognized it. "Hell, that's just the general informed-consent form," he said. "Everyone signs it whether they're going to have an appendectomy or brain surgery. So what?"

"Mr. Anthony," Steinhardt said, turning with exaggerated movement toward the Coit Hill administrator. "Have you read section six of paragraph ten of your form lately?" He didn't wait for Anthony to answer. "Let me refresh your memory. 'Should a complex and unforeseen problem arise, I, the undersigned, do hereby grant the physician in charge to use whatever drug, device, or procedure is at his disposal and that he believes, according to his best judgment, may be reasonable to use in the case of the above-named patient.' In other words, Coit Hill's consent form, we believe, indirectly provides for the use of what might be construed as an experimental process. Certainly under emergency circumstances . . ."

"So you have an informed-consent form, so what?" Anthony said. "From what I know about that evening, no one even had time to get the family to sign."

"Oh, you're quite wrong about that, Mr. Anthony. If I read correctly this name under the space where someone from the hospital has to sign, I believe that a Miss Cluny went to the trouble of seeing to it that the family signed this consent form. In any case, given the provisions of what we consider a key paragraph in that form and given the state of Dr. Kirk's work with his artificial blood formula, we are prepared to argue in a court of law that under the circumstances—namely, that no surgeon would answer Dr. Kirk's summons to come to the aid of the boy—Dr. Kirk was indeed justified in trying to use his formula. We are prepared to allow a jury to decide the question."

"Fine. Let us for the moment assume that a jury will accept that the section in the informed-consent form constitutes acceptance of a highly experimental procedure," Cummings said. "We still don't quite see the necessity for taking up a court's valuable time, not to mention all of ours, in a case that is otherwise cut and dried."

"Cut and dried how, Mr. Cummings?" Steinhardt sounded as though he sincerely wanted Cummings to educate him on something he had missed.

"Cut and dried in that Dr. Kirk's artificial blood solution brought on cardiac arrest and the boy's premature death."

"On what authority do you come to that conclusion?"

"I don't know that we need that much authority," Anthony interjected. "The facts seem to be fairly clear. Not a minute after Dr. Kirk injected his formula, the boy went into cardiac arrest."

Steinhardt laughed. "You people could give lessons in railroad justice. Get off it! You had this boy on the ropes and you just decided to cut yourselves the best deal you could to protect yourselves. You just weren't going to let the facts get in the way, were you?"

"Roger, I appreciate your talents as an attorney as well as anyone," Cole said. "But come on. Dr. Kirk must have given you enough of the truth to let you decide that you have a basically indefensible action here."

"You mean the administration of the artificial blood?"

"Of course the administration of the blood! What the hell else are we talking about?"

"The administration of the blood may have been indefensible. But that does not mean that the blood killed the boy. And if in some way the administration of the compound was contrary to procedure, we still have that fact that the administration of the compound and the death are two separate issues. We only have to win one of them, Joyce, and you know that as well as I do."

"And you are prepared to go to court to prove that Dr. Kirk's artificial blood did not play a role in the death of the patient?" This time it was White who came into the conversation.

"That should not be terribly difficult to establish," Dr. Creighton said.

Phil Dorr, who had until now followed the sparring among the lawyers and the administrators halfheartedly, turned to the pathologist with interest. "You have reason to argue that the artificial blood, specifically an immune response to the blood, did not contribute to the boy's death?"

"Substantial reason and it is based on very recent research with artificial blood compounds. Remember that the patient died just a few minutes after the administration of the blood. Until just recently, most pathologists would have told you that the quick death meant that some specific cells that are the signs of an anaphylactoid, an immune, response if you will, would not have had time to form. Therefore, until now, any supposition that a death may have been a response to the artificial blood would have had to be equivocal at best. But recent work at the University of Minnesota shows that in experimental animals anaphylactoid deaths from an artificial blood compound are very clearly associated with the accumulation of clumped white cells in the pulmonary capillaries within a very few minutes. I have looked at slides of the patient's lung tissue at the medical examiner's office. There are absolutely no signs of a capillary infiltration. In other words, the death was not due to an immune response to the blood."

"Then, doctor, if in your opinion the artificial blood did not cause death, why did the kid die?" Anthony asked.

"My opinion doesn't quite matter since the pathology report was quite clear on that. He died of prolonged hypovolemia."

"I'm sorry, doctor," Cummings cut in. "That word was not covered in my high school biology class."

"He died of severe blood loss, Mr. Cummings," Creighton answered. "The patient apparently sustained a severe blow to the liver and extensive damage to other organs, all which resulted in an exsanguinating hemorrhage."

"Dr. Creighton, did you also study the medical records Coit Hill supplied the medical examiner?" Steinhardt asked.

"Yes, of course."

"And what did you think of the medical care?"

"What's the point of that question?" Cummings interrupted again. "Let's confine ourselves to the immediate issues."

"I think the quality of care at Coit Hill is very much at issue here."

Cummings sat back in his chair.

"Insofar as I can see, the quality of care in the emergency room was heroic. Certainly all that Dr. Kirk could have done for the young man was done. However, given the extent of the damage to the liver and other organs, without timely surgical intervention, the patient was doomed. No amount of fluid replacement could have sustained him indefinitely."

"Without implying disrespect for Dr. Creighton," Cole said, "these are matters on which there might be different opinions." She turned to White, Cummings, and Anthony. "In any case, with Dr. Kirk determined to contest the matter, the settlement we discussed is now moot."

Cummings shifted himself back toward the table and glared at Steinhardt. "You really are prepared to take this sham defense to court?"

"And we are also prepared to go to court on the other five malpractice suits you filed. Not to mention the complaint we will file against you with the bar."

Cummings flushed visibly. "What complaint with the bar?"

"Unprofessional behavior," Steinhardt answered. "Soliciting the lawsuits you filed against Dr. Kirk. And when we are through with that, we'll see you in civil court on my client's slander and libel suit."

"You're mad."

"Am I really? You haven't seen anything yet. I would strongly recommend that you, Joyce, advise the University that it will quite likely have to answer in court for the illegal fashion in which it dismissed Dr. Kirk from his various positions." Steinhardt was rolling. In spite of themselves, his opponents were mesmerized by his voice. "And I would recommend that both you and Mr. Cummings suggest to your clients the name of a law firm well versed in antitrust law because the University and Coit Hill had better be prepared to defend against a complaint that will be filed next week with the appropriate authorities, that they engaged in an illegal act to restrain trade by secretly agreeing on the manner in which trauma and other patients are to be divided between the two institutions."

They all started talking at Steinhardt at once, but Cummings's voice cut through. "Steinhardt, this sort of approach may work with the other cockamamy cases you take up, but it's not going to work here, with us. We are not going to help you bluff your client out of the mess he's in."

Steinhardt stood. "Harrison, if you think we are bluffing, you're perfectly welcome to call us on it. In the meantime, as they say, we'll be in touch." As he walked out, Allan, who had been virtually forgotten in the course of the debate, scrambled to get on his feet to keep up with his attorney. Creighton smiled at the group, slowly pushed himself out of his chair, and followed suit.

Before anyone could say anything, Dorr bolted out after the trio. Half trotting, half walking down the corridor, he caught up with Steinhardt, Kirk, and Creighton just before they reached the bank of elevators. He reached out and took hold of Allan's arm.

Allan turned around and faced the man whom he had for so long considered his mentor. In that first instant his eyes locked with Dorr's. The older man's gaze was immensely sad.

"Son, is all this your idea?"

At the sound of his voice, Steinhardt and Creighton, who had been walking just slightly ahead of Allan, stopped. Steinhardt took two steps back. "If you have anything to say . . ."

Allan held up his hand. "It's all right. Is this all my idea? What do you think, Phil?"

Dorr, with his hand still around Allan's biceps, was agonizing, wanting to speak, not knowing really what to say, in what direction to take the conversation. "Allan, it will cause such a terrible mess."

"You mean a mess greater than you tried to make out of my life?" Allan roughly wrenched himself out of Dorr's grasp. "You almost had me convinced, Phil, that all of this, as you put it, was my doing, that I had screwed up so badly that I was destroying the University, the system, what have you. It was stupid of me to feel that way, but not for the reasons you think. It was stupid because if I was guilty of anything it was for caring too much for the people who I thought depended on me. And I was guilty of thinking that preventing a nineteen-year-old kid from bleeding to death in front of my eyes was more important than anything else in the world. But that was all I was—and am—guilty of. If you're going to punish me for that, then you're going to have to pay a price for the privilege."

"I'm sure we can work something out."

Allan sensed that Steinhardt was about to interfere again, so again he waved him off.

"Now things can be worked out? Why now, all of a sudden, Phil? Because you find you may have cast your lot with the wrong people? Because now you have something at stake too?"

"Walter," Dorr said, turning to the pathologist. "You've been through battles like this. . . ."

"And you want me to talk him out of it?" The old man smiled indulgently at Dorr. "No, Phil. The boy is right, you know. It's a battle he's fighting correctly."

Dorr shook his head, turned, and walked back to the conference room. Allan watched him for a moment. He felt a sharp grief and he was tempted to go after Dorr, to tell him that yes, they could talk. Instead, he turned to his colleagues. "I'm hungry," he said. "Let's go eat."

"Is Julie joining us?" Creighton asked.

"Well, she said she would try to meet us at the restaurant if she's able to leave the office in time."

Julie took her customary last look around the office and walked briskly to the reception desk, hoping the security guard would walk her to the car. But the old man was not around, probably, Julie thought, making his rounds through the building. She considered waiting for him. But, eager to meet Allan and the others, she walked to the front door and peered out at the walkways and the parking lot, then decided to make her way to the car by herself.

With a quick glance over her shoulder to make sure the guard had not returned, she walked out. The early evening was quiet and if somewhat cool, nevertheless comfortable. Soothed by the air, she started to think about her Allan and the evening ahead.

The man's rough voice shook her out of her reverie. "You're Julie McDonough, right?"

She wheeled, almost falling in the process. An old-style Navy pea coat covered the man's torso. Though he was bald, his face was covered by a closely cropped beard. His nose was broad and flat. His eyes forced her to look into them.

"Don't be afraid," he said, talking in a low voice, not taking his eyes off her. "I'm not here to hurt you. Just keep walking. I want to talk to you about your friend, Dr. Kirk, and the way he's been carrying on lately."

Julie managed to look past him, hoping to find the security guard. "The old man's gone to check on the stiffs, Miss McDonough," the man said, and pointed for her to turn around.

She followed the unspoken order. The man grasped her elbow. "Just listen and I'll get out of your way. Your friend is really something, Miss McDonough. These days it's nice to see someone that committed, someone who is so sure of what he wants. But you know, it's one thing to be committed, it's another to step on people's toes just to get your own way. People don't like to be stepped on, Miss McDonough. You and Dr. Kirk have to understand that important people especially don't like it when someone starts to step all over them."

Julie's legs weakened. The man seemed to sense her reaction because he tightened his grip as if to give her support. "What is it you want?" she asked, barely managing to get the words out.

"I don't want anything from you, Miss McDonough. I'd just like to give you some advice that you can pass on. When important people get upset, accidents happen. I'm worried about Dr. Kirk. He's too good a doctor to lose. But he's pushing too hard, Miss McDonough. He's pushing too hard." There was a short pause. "Talk to him. Maybe you can talk some sense into him, you're an intelligent girl. You're smart enough a young lady to make him see he's taken things far enough. If I were you and if you care about him, I wouldn't let this continue."

They had reached the car. The man looked around. "Think about what I said, Miss McDonough." He nodded and walked briskly away.

She leaned against the car, her breath coming in short gasps. Struggling to stay on her feet and shaking, she reached into her bag to fish out her keys. With every movement an effort, she inserted the ignition key and turned it. She heard only a slight click. She tried again. The car did not respond. Fighting the instinct to scream, she reached beneath the steering wheel and pulled on the hood release. When she lifted the hood and looked at the engine she saw that the battery was gone.

The fat manila envelope was sitting on Allan's doorstep when he, Steinhardt, and Creighton returned from the dinner.

"That was a damned good meal," Steinhardt said as Allan picked up the envelope and studied it. "Too bad Julie didn't make it."

"Yeah," Allan said, turning the envelope over again. "I guess she just got tied up at work." He flicked on a light and headed for the couch. "She'll catch up to us here, I guess." He tore open the envelope and pulled out a thick sheaf of papers held together by a rubber band. While the others watched, he shuffled through the packet.

Allan looked up, a somewhat dazed expression on his face. "It's a copy of the mayor's medical records. E.R. notes, O.R. notes, an X ray, autopsy results. Everything."

Creighton, having heard the word "mayor," came over. "Do you know who sent it?"

"I have a suspicion it's Everett Huntington," Allan answered. "It has to be." He turned his attention back to the records. Suddenly he whacked them on the coffee table in front of him. "We have them by the short hairs," he said, triumph in his voice. "We got them by the very, very short hairs."

Creighton started to say something, but was interrupted by the door bell. Allan leapt up to open the door.

"I can tell you were expecting someone else," Younger said, as he walked in.

"Julie."

"Well, sorry to let you down," Younger said, noting for the first time that Creighton and Steinhardt were present. "You got in touch with them. Have they been any help?"

"Thanks. They might be saving my life." Allan put his hand on Younger's shoulder. "Stick around for a while and we might be able to tell you about the mayor's murder."

"We don't know that the mayor was murdered," Creighton said quickly. "All we have is some medical records that may tell us how he died."

"And that he didn't have to die in the first place," Allan interjected, unrelenting.

"We don't know that either," Creighton responded quietly. "At least not yet."

"Is there a chance I can use whatever you find for tomorrow's paper?" Younger asked.

"Why don't we wait and see what there is in there before we decide?" Creighton said.

"Fair enough. Will you go on the record?" Younger asked, looking pointedly at Creighton.

"Yes, naturally. You know I don't hide my opinions behind a cloak of anonymity."

For an hour, while Younger watched television and Steinhardt buried himself in the first draft of a brief he was preparing to file in the biker malpractice suit, Allan and Creighton studied the material in the folders line by line. Occasionally, Allan would ask the pathologist something or Creighton would hand a sheet of paper over to Allan for his perusal.

Toward the end of the second sitcom he had drifted into, Younger looked over to the kitchen and saw Allan staring off into space, apparently thinking something out. Creighton was almost finished with the fourth folder. Younger punched the Off button on the remote-control panel in his lap. "Well?" he called out. "Has the jury reached a decision?"

Creighton stood up and walked to the sink for a glass of water. "It's a tough case," he said as he put the glass back down on the counter.

A look of disappointment crossed Younger's face, and Creighton laughed. "Oh, don't worry. You've still got a story. But it certainly is not the case of out-and-out negligence you might be wishing for."

"It's not?" Younger and Allan spoke in unison.

"I don't think it is. On its face, the case was mishandled. The record and particularly the X ray indicate that the mayor suffered a pneumothorax. Strictly speaking, it should have been recognized in the emergency room and if it had been, a chest tube would have made a major difference. But it was not. And, to make matters seem worse, the damage to the lungs was not noted in the operating room either."

Allan pivoted. "Why be so cautious? It's not some theoretical problem we're talking about here. They simply did not discover the injuries they should have and as a result the mayor died. Period. They murdered the man and then they covered it up."

"I can see, young man, how it is that you get yourself into so much hot water," Creighton said. "In any case, it doesn't help matters to say they 'murdered' the mayor, as if he had been on the road to recovery after surgery and they had yanked his IVs. At best you can say that he did not receive optimal care. And whether or not Coit Hill 'covered up' anything would be for a grand jury to determine."

"And if you were summoned before the grand jury, what would you recommend on that score?" Younger asked.

"That is certainly not within my province. Looking at the

situation from the most kindly viewpoint, however, I would say the hospital people panicked and released an inappropriate explanation for the mayor's death."

"Oh, bullshit!" Allan said, slapping the tabletop.

Creighton looked squarely at Allan. "You cannot ignore the fact that the mayor was in the operating room within fifteen minutes of admission. That is a time lapse many a trauma center could envy."

Allan, wide-eyed, came around the table toward Creighton. "I don't believe this! Are you saying that, based on those records, you would tell a grand jury that the mayor received commendable care?"

"Careful of the words you choose, Allan. I did not say he received commendable care, nor did I even remotely hint that."

"All right, I know now what you would not say. What would you say?"

"I would say that the mayor's death was unacceptable."

"I think I'm confused," Younger broke in.

"If our young friend here would allow me a few uninterrupted sentences, you would not be." He glanced over at Allan, who now made a point of turning away and rummaging through the refrigerator.

"A trauma case can be mismanaged at many different levels," Creighton continued. "Obviously the most dramatic way is to bring a patient into an emergency room where little or nothing is done, where the patient is simply allowed to bleed to death in an hour. The next step up—or down, depending on your point of view—is the case in which a patient is brought into an emergency room where he gets some help, but not enough. He is monitored, but not often enough, he is given fluids or blood, but not in sufficient quantities, he is given one chest tube instead of two.

"On to the next level. We can imagine an emergency room where the physician or physicians on duty are competent, do everything right, but then have to watch their patient bleed to death anyway because they cannot get the right surgeons to come in."

"But that is what happened here!" Allan called out.

"In a sense it did, yes. The first man or two they called did not respond. But a surgeon and an anesthesiologist were in the O.R. by the time the mayor arrived there. And that is precisely my point and one you consistently fail to make. What ultimately determines a patient's outcome may not be emergency-room care, may not be consultant response time, but the expertise of the people treating the patient. What a trauma center offers, above all, are people who see so many cases of trauma that their response to even the most terrible and complex of cases is automatic and sure. What was missing in the mayor's case was expertise, expertise gained from seeing the same thing over and over again."

"That's not the sort of thing people understand," Allan said slowly. "It's not the kind of explanation that is going to make the public finally sit up and take notice."

"Maybe not," Creighton answered. "But in this case, at least, that's what you are stuck with. If you are depending on the mayor's death to advance the case for redesigning San Francisco's hospital system so that there is only one, committed trauma center, you're going to have to take what you can get. And what you can get in this case is that Coit Hill blew it because they just weren't experienced enough."

"So if Coit Hill were the only trauma center in the county, that would be all right?" Younger asked.

"Not necessarily," Creighton continued. "If Coit Hill is allowed to become a self-designated trauma center, if any hospital becomes a self-designated center, it may get enough cases of trauma to keep the hospital administration happy. But as long as there is no organized system in San Francisco that channels all trauma cases to that trauma center, hundreds of other cases will go to other hospitals. The doctors at the self-designated center, in this case Coit Hill, will never gain the experience they need to save someone's life in fifteen minutes, X rays and a million pieces of sophisticated equipment notwithstanding.

"In any case, I don't think that is much of a concern at the moment. Whether you call it a cover-up or not, the fact is that they did not come clean about the death when it happened. I would guess that after Sam writes his story, the hospital and its administration are going to be in plenty of hot water with the authorities and would not be able to make much of a bid to become a trauma center, much less the only one for the city."

For the third time Younger looked at his watch. "Shit! I missed the morning edition." He turned to Allan. "Does anyone else have this?"

"Not that I know of."

"You going to tell anyone?"

"Sam, I owe you," Allan said. "When can you get it in?"

"I'll go to the office now and write it. But the earliest I can make is the Wednesday edition that will hit the streets about ten-thirty Tuesday night. Anthony and his friends can read the story after they leave the meeting of the Joint Committee."

"The one the supervisors ordered after your story on the study ran?" Allan asked.

"That's the one. The letter from the chairman of the Board of Supervisors to the committee practically orders it to come up with some kind of a system. I guess the phones have been ringing off the hook at the supes' offices. There is a good deal of public pressure building up for the county to do something."

Steinhardt watched Younger leave the apartment, then clapped enthusiastically in Allan's direction. "Congratulations, Allan, it's all coming together for you. By tomorrow night, Anthony should be on his way out of town."

"I'd like to believe that, but somehow I doubt it. I'm sure that Huntington sent those records and I should be grateful, I guess. But I think I should go see him and find out what else he knows, and if he'll go public."

"Anonymously sending you the records is one thing," Steinhardt said. "But you think he'll go public? What for? He's got nothing to gain."

"Maybe not, but I've got to convince him. I've got to get him to tell people about the kind of trauma center Anthony runs. If he does that, if he gives the public an insider's view of the way that megalomaniac works, then maybe Anthony won't be able to squirm his way out of it." Allan threw on a jacket. "Let yourselves out," he said. "I want to get going."

He strode to the door and opened it. Standing on the other side, her finger poised at the doorbell, was Julie.

"Hey! Where have you been?" he asked, then kept talking without giving her a chance to answer. "I'm on my way to see Everett Huntington. He sent over the mayor's medical records. I want to talk to him about going public with—"

"Allan," Julie whispered. "Please don't."

He scrutinized her face. "Jesus! What's the matter?"

"Allan, I'm scared," she managed before she began to cry.

16

Allan stopped at the door leading into the room where the Joint Committee for Emergency Services was meeting and waited for Julie, who had stopped to take a drink from a water fountain.

"Get a load of this," he said to her as she approached.

Julie looked at the sign on the door. "What is that supposed to mean: 'In Executive Session'?"

"It means just that," said Younger, who had come up behind them. "They have probably found some excuse to meet behind closed doors. I'd guess they'll open it up in a few minutes, though. They announced this as a public meeting."

Allan stared at the locked door. "I'd sure like to know what is going on in there."

Younger looked around, then pointed to another door a few feet away. "Let's see what's in there."

Julie and Allan followed Younger into the empty room. To their right several hundred chairs were neatly stacked next to a conventional wall. The wall to their left was a ceiling-to-floor folding vinyl divider.

"The reporter's best friend," Younger said, "the accordion

room divider." He laughed at Allan and Julie's quizzical look. "Okay, say a union is on the verge of calling a strike and they hold a meeting in a hotel ballroom, for example. If they don't need all that space, they ask for the divider to be drawn so they don't have to pay as much rental. Along come the reporters, but they are barred from the meeting. Enterprising journalists that we are, we just go to the other side of the divider and listen in. Pull up chairs, folks, and let's hear what our friends are up to."

Julie cast Allan a worried look. "We've got enough intrigue already."

"Julie, are you still worried?"

"You know I am."

Younger looked from one to the other. "Worried about what?" Allan told him about the man who had approached Julie, then turned to Julie. "Sweetheart, nothing is going to happen. Anthony is just playing games, that's all. He may be determined to have his way with his trauma center, but he's not a murderer."

"I'm not worried about me. It's you I'm concerned about. I don't want anything to happen to you."

Allan gathered Julie into his arms and held her tightly for a minute. "I'll tell you what," he said after a moment. "If Huntington doesn't show up, I'll just sit there nice and quiet when we go in. If the committee people want to question me about our study, I'll answer and nothing more. I won't say a thing about the mayor's death. They can read about it in the paper later tonight."

"And if Huntington does come, you're still going to insist on airing the mayor's case here?"

"Yes, that is still the optimal way."

"Why not just let Sam's story take care of Anthony?"

"Because it should be nailed down as tightly as possible. Anthony has a thousand ways of wiggling out of tight spots, and the only way to neutralize him is to have Huntington air, before witnesses, what happened at Coit. And he has to do it before Anthony has a chance to put pressure on him to rescind his story or soften it." Allan stopped for breath. "Anyway, Huntington told me that Anthony had fired him, but he sent me copies of the records because he had already gotten fed up with Coit, not to get even with Anthony. But he also said he could only go so far, meaning that he wasn't going to go public. Come on, let's see if we can hear anything through that wall."

"Al, surely you're not serious," someone was saying. "After the stout way in which we have defended the hospital system in this county, you want to say that Kirk is right?"

"I'm perfectly serious. What we cannot afford to do is to allow the offensive to pass over completely on this. I say we announce that the Kirk study is revealing and that we have to move to act on it. We tell the county health officer that he should conduct an investigation to ascertain the extent to which Kirk's study is correct."

"And, in the meantime, if we do nothing the press will scream that we are ignoring the fact that thousands die," another voice said.

"But we won't be doing nothing," Anthony said, almost managing to sound triumphant. "We will announce that until the health officer's study is in, Coit Hill will provide the trauma service the county needs."

"How convenient, Al," someone said. "And the other institutions in the county are supposed to stand aside while you siphon off a goodly portion of their emergency-room business?"

"All right, then let's do this. Have the hospital council write the criteria the paramedics in the field will use to determine if someone is injured critically enough to be diverted to our trauma center. This committee can set up a review board to audit Coit Hill's admissions every six months to see if we're stealing patients who are less seriously injured and could go to conventional emergency rooms."

"Al, it won't work."

"It has to work! If we don't do it this way, the field will be open to Kirk, the supervisors will bring in out-of-county experts to set up a trauma system, and we'll lose complete control of the matter."

"I don't think we can convince the other hospitals in this area that they should buy your plan, Al, no matter what criteria you write or what kind of a watchdog committee you set up. I can't think of one administrator who would just step aside for you like that."

"Okay, fine, they want part of the action, we can give it to them," Anthony said, his voice tight. "How many hospitals in the county do you think would want to deal with trauma patients?"

"There are several other hospitals, including the University, that would be willing to set up some sort of trauma service, provided it didn't cost them too much," a new voice said.

"All right, let's set up a rotating trauma system. Every fourth week, each hospital takes its turn receiving trauma patients."

Allan leaned close to Julie and Younger. "What a wheeler," he whispered. "He knows darned well what will happen. After six months the other hospitals will look at their books and they'll see that the trouble of doing trauma one week a month isn't worth it, either in aggravation or money, so they'll start dropping out of the rotation. The end result will be the same, Coit Hill will be the sole trauma center by default."

". . . not to mention the fact," Anthony was continuing, "that there is one very good reason to go along with this. If you allow others to tell us where trauma centers should be, the next thing you know they'll be telling you which hospital should have exclusive rights to set up a neonatal intensive-care unit, which one should do all the heart surgery in San Francisco. We can't relinquish our independence like that. We have to draw the line here!"

For a moment there was a silence. "Al, it's getting close to seven-thirty," a voice finally said. "Let's open this thing up and see if anyone is going to show up."

Younger, Julie, and Allan scurried out of the room. Allan scanned the hall. "Huntington isn't here, so I guess he isn't going to show up, the bastard."

Julie closed her eyes in relief. But when she opened them, the first thing she saw beyond Allan's shoulder was Everett Huntington walking purposefully down the hall toward them.

"You were right, Allan," Everett Huntington said. "What do we do now?"

Allan grinned broadly and for an answer threw open the door

to the meeting room. Propelling Huntington forward, he walked his colleague toward the committee, keeping his eyes on Anthony, relishing the alarm that was spreading over the administrator's face.

They lifted their glasses in a silent toast, then sipped the champagne they had ordered at the first semirespectable bar they had found.

"Everett," Allan said, "thanks again for coming. I was pretty sure you wouldn't show up."

"When you left last night I was pretty sure I wasn't going to."

"Then what changed your mind?" Younger asked.

"Lying in bed, thinking about the kid Fedder operated on, thinking about the way his folks were looking at their son in the recovery room. It just hurt to think what it would have been like if the little bugger had died on me. It came over me that I couldn't allow that to happen again, that if I didn't follow up on the course I had taken when I gave you the records, it could happen again. I said a few prayers and came to meet you."

Julie poured them all another glass of champagne. "Do you think they were serious?"

"About making me head of a subcommittee to devise the trauma system? I guess so. But it just doesn't seem real."

"I think they realized that with Anthony discredited now, they had no choice," Younger said. "They had to show that they weren't just Anthony's puppets. So asking you to set up the process to evaluate the applications hospitals submit and to set up the system to evaluate the new trauma center was the least they could do. And besides, they may be stubborn and may be more interested in their own welfare than the public's, but they are not stupid. I guess they figure that at the very least they are better off having someone from the local medical community develop a trauma plan than possibly having the Board of Supervisors call in consultants from outside the county to do it. This way the docs and the hospitals still have some small chance of influencing the way things come out."

Julie drank from her glass. "In a sense you were lucky, weren't you?"

"How so?"

"That Anthony tried to fudge what happened to the mayor. If he had come clean he could still have had a shot at building his empire."

"Probably. But I don't know if I would call it luck. That megalomaniac got so wrapped up in this trauma business, he wanted it so badly at any cost that eventually he would have made a mistake and it would have come crashing down around him. Without a commitment from his people all he had was an empty shell. Any little thing would eventually have destroyed it, and him. Come on, let's go find a *Telegraph* and see what the story about the mayor looks like on the front page."

They started to leave, but Allan stopped them. "Which reminds me," he said, hoisting a glass toward Younger. "Thanks for the help. I know I was angry about those early stories you wrote, but I certainly couldn't have done as much without your coverage."

Anthony sat statue still and let his eyes roam, for probably the fifth time in the last twenty minutes, over the front-page story in the *Telegraph*. Out of the corner of his eye he could see the eight buttons on his telephone console. They had remained lit since he came in earlier in the morning. If one light did go out, it was only a second or two until it was on again. Time and again he heard his secretary tell the reporters calling from across the state as well as from local news outlets that he was busy in meetings and was not available for comment. There were, to boot, reporters, camera crews, and photographers stationed on the approaches to the hospital, in the emergency waiting room, in the hall outside his office. He had managed to sneak into the hospital only because no one had thought of covering the docking platform where the delivery trucks left the hospital's supplies. The only one who had apparently not tried to get through to him was Cummings, the person he wanted most to talk with.

As Anthony started to read the article once more, the second phone on his desk—his private line—gave out its muted ring. He snatched the phone off the hook.

"I was just beginning to wonder when you'd get around to me," Anthony said through gritted teeth.

"My dear fellow, I've had to sneak out of my office to get away from the phone calls from the nation's journalists. Be thankful I'm talking to you now."

"What are we going to do?"

"That's a bit difficult to say right now."

"What are you waiting for? A revelation from Melvin Belli? What the hell is wrong with you?"

Cummings ignored the insults. "What I mean is that the newspaper story per se is only part of your difficulties at the moment. The most pressing problem is likely to be the district attorney."

"The D.A.? What does the D.A. have to do with this?"

"Rowlands hasn't been in touch with you?" Cummings's voice was quiet now.

"I haven't been taking calls."

"He wants you, and me, to come down to his office for an interview. There is every likelihood that there will be a grand jury investigation."

"God Almighty! You—they couldn't be serious."

"I'm afraid that I, and they, probably are. District attorneys lead grand juries around by the nose. And like every D.A. in the world, Rowlands is politically ambitious, not to mention a member of the late mayor's party. If he thinks he can get Creighton to repeat his interpretation of the records in court, and there is no reason to think he won't, and if he can get at least one other expert to back Creighton in his analysis of what happened to the mayor, he'll go for some kind of an indictment, whether on the death itself or on the way the pneumothorax was expunged from the records."

"That shit-eating Kirk!"

"Oh, I wouldn't be so fast to blame Kirk, Al. He is only doing what comes naturally. He got those records from someone else, and my guess is that it's someone you pushed too far."

"He got them from Huntington, that sorry son of a bitch. I'll get him. He violated the state's patient-privacy laws and I've got a contact in the attorney general's office in Sacramento. I'll—"

"Forget it, Al. I doubt the attorney general's office would move on that, especially if the grand jury returns an indictment. Huntington got his pound of flesh; don't aggravate it by making him look like another hero."

Anthony said nothing.

"Al, are you there? There's one more thing."

"Yes, I'm here."

"The board of directors' meeting . . ."

"Mother of God! That's at three today," Anthony cried, bending his head closer toward the phone. "Harrison, get them to call it off. I can't face that today."

"I doubt seriously that I could do that, Al, especially today. But you had better prepare a damned good explanation for what happened with the mayor."

Though he had never taken a drink before lunch, Anthony went to his liquor cabinet and poured himself a Scotch and water that was tall even by his standards. Drink in hand, he returned to his desk and pulled out the copy of the mayor's records that he had been keeping. Sipping from the drink, he went through the folders page by page. By the time he had finished the drink and his review, he had convinced himself again that he had nothing to worry about, that no one could have saved the mayor. Satisfied, he looked again for the hospital pathologist's report, then searched through the top drawer in his desk until he found a thick felt marker. Careful to be neat, he underlined the two paragraphs in the pathologist's report that discussed the mayor's heart-disease history, then asked his secretary to make enough copies for everyone on the executive committee. As for the missing references to the pneumothorax, he muttered to himself, it wouldn't be too hard to pin that on a panicky Huntington, trying to save his own rear end.

He dialed Sherman Harper's number, hoping to ask him to attend the board meeting with him to discuss the mayor's heart disease. Harper's office told him that the cardiac surgeon had gone into the operating room at seven in the morning and, because he had scheduled three procedures in succession, was not likely to emerge until mid-afternoon. Anthony dialed the operating room, but Harper refused to take the call.

To the devil with Harper too, Anthony fumed. He had always been his own best lobbyist, especially under pressure. He found the list with the names and telephone numbers of each of the board members and began to call. He reached only two and they politely told him that they would discuss nothing with him until later in the day. At ten minutes to three, finally convinced that he had run out of options, he asked the hospital security guard to help him get to the board meeting by running interference for him through the reporters who were still camped in the hall.

He had used the brief walk to the board room to pump himself up and now, as he came in, he walked briskly to his place at the long oval table. Because these meetings were held only once a month, the board's agenda was always heavily laden. As a result, Anthony was forced to come with a half dozen or so folders, each one related to the topics that had to be discussed. Before he had left his office for this meeting, he had made sure that he had with him the folders that corresponded to the agenda that he had drawn up and distributed three days before the *Telegraph*'s story on the mayor's death broke. He was going to show the assembled group that, as far as he was concerned, it would be business as usual. He put the folders down, smiled, and greeted each member of the board by name. It disturbed him only slightly to note that at least three members of the board refused to look him squarely in the eye as he swept his gaze around the table. The one director who met his gaze straight on and held it was Richard Marden. Anthony tried hard to see in those eyes a hint that Marden still supported him. But in the man's cool stare he could sense only that the hinges holding the gallows' trapdoor were oiled and ready to give way quickly.

Anthony plowed on with his plan to treat the meeting as routine. "Before we take up the misleading story in today's *Telegraph*, there are some important items on the agenda that we—"

"The story on the front page of the paper, Al, is at the top of our agenda," Marden said, his voice slow and measured.

Anthony pushed the folders away. "All right, then, let's get that out of the way so we can get to the more pressing matters."

Marden would not relent. "The mayor's death is the only pressing matter, Al."

Anthony sighed heavily. He reached for the pile of folders and drew them back toward him. He picked out the thickest one, third from the top. He opened it and took out several packets, each containing several pieces of paper stapled together, and gave each member of the board one of the packets.

"What I am distributing to you is a summary of the information we have, including our pathologist's report, on the medical treatment accorded the mayor in this institution. As you read it over, I am sure that you will see that we have nothing to be ashamed of. The mayor could not have received better care in any hospital in this county."

Not one of the people sitting at the table with him made a move to read the papers he had distributed and Marden, it seemed to Anthony, made a point of pushing away the set in front of him.

"What is your interpretation of the article in this morning's newspaper?" Marden asked.

"The story is wrong."

"As simple as that?"

"Yes," Anthony retorted. "All Dr. Creighton had to go on were medical records. I grant you they were the same records we have here, the same records summarized in the material before you. But there is a crucial difference. Dr. Creighton did not see the patient. He did not deal, as our physicians did, with the mayor in the flesh. Medical records are well and good. But if you haven't dealt with the patient, you have no right to say what the doctors who did deal with him should or should not have done."

"I don't think Dr. Creighton would agree," Marden said. He was obviously talking as the board's spokesman.

"He's a pathologist, someone who works with microscopes and cadavers. The man has never seen a patient with a bad cold," Anthony persisted. "What can he possibly know about what care should be extended, particularly in a pressured situation like this one?"

"Al, it seems to me that you are not being very forthright, or perhaps not very realistic. Dr. Creighton has an impeccable reputation as a pathologist in this community." It was Francine Normans, the sole woman on the board. She had been a nurse before she married a young man who had been hospitalized at Coit Hill for an appendectomy. After the marriage she had stopped work and had dedicated herself to her marriage and family. But, still interested in medicine and Coit Hill, she later became one of the hospital's most enthusiastic volunteers. As a reward for her many efforts, she had, two years earlier, been appointed to the board of directors.

"I am not impugning Dr. Creighton's reputation, Mrs. Normans. I'm only saying that no one can judge a case just on the basis of records. You have to be able to look at the patient."

"And you believe that Dr. Creighton, knowing that, would be foolish enough to stick his neck out in a major way?" Marden asked.

Anthony leaned back in his chair. "The man is what, seventy, seventy-five, and retired for a good eight years? Maybe he has lost touch with the realities of medicine."

"That is totally unnecessary, Mr. Anthony," Francine Normans reprimanded. "Dr. Creighton's standing in the community is not based solely on his reputation, but on his continuing medical activities as well. You'll not help your cause or this hospital's if you insist on uncalled-for slurs on those who differ with you."

"In any case," interrupted one of the more recent appointees to the board, the general manager of San Francisco's educational television station, Zachary Scott, "Creighton is not the only one mentioned in the Younger story. Dr. Kirk agrees with the pathologist's assessment."

"With all due respect, Mr. Scott, I don't think Dr. Kirk's opinion is worth..." Anthony stopped short of using the scatalogical word that almost escaped. Still stinging from the earlier rebuke, he took care to measure his words. "Dr. Kirk is obviously biased against this institution because of its efforts to establish itself as a trauma center. And I don't have to remind you that his judgments as a physician are questionable as well."

"His judgments as a researcher may be questionable, Mr. Anthony," Scott pressed on. "I'm not sure I would question his values as a doctor. From what I have heard from friends on the University's board of directors, his dedication as a physician is beyond reproach."

"In any case, Al, what is and is not in the newspaper is, at this point, irrelevant to this board," Marden interjected.

Anthony blinked. "I'm not sure I follow you. I thought this morning's story was what we are talking about."

"I'm sorry if I confused you. What I meant to say was that for the moment we are not entirely dependent on Dr. Creighton or Dr. Kirk's opinions in the matter. It doesn't really matter whether Dr. Creighton was here or not and whether or not Dr. Kirk has credibility."

"I'm sorry, maybe I am not following well what is happening here, but just exactly what does matter?"

"Two things. One, that you forced members of this hospital's staff to falsify the mayor's records so that there would be no mention of the critical lung wound. Two, that earlier this morning each one of us received, by messenger, a detailed analysis of the care the mayor received. The conclusion of that analysis—which, unlike yours, does contain the X-ray report on the lung puncture—also is that the mayor's life might have been saved if the people treating him had appreciated the fact that he had a lung wound. The report was signed by Dr. Everett Huntington."

"Dr. Huntington is not exactly a disinterested party either," Anthony said, sliding back toward the table. "He's getting back at us because I fired him earlier this week because—"

"We are well aware of why you fired Dr. Huntington, Mr. Anthony," Mrs. Normans interrupted. "And we believe he acted honorably in doing everything he could to save that child's life. Which brings us to yet another point."

Anthony studied her and suddenly understood that she was the enemy, that this woman who had filled her long daytime hours with incessant volunteer efforts in behalf of the hospital was, in all probability, the leader in this effort to court-martial him. She cared about Coit Hill, it was evident to Anthony; she believed profoundly in its sanctity, in its value to the community, in its importance as a San Francisco institution. She had become a true believer in Coit Hill's cause. And now, Anthony knew, she saw him as the person who could be responsible for Coit Hill's fall from grace. It would not be something for which she would stand still.

"Mr. Anthony?" she said now.

"Yes, I'm sorry, Mrs. Normans. You were saying something about another point?"

"You were very persuasive in convincing us that this hospital could serve as a trauma center. We approved the expenditure of millions of dollars, not just to outfit Coit Hill with a helicopter service, but to expand the emergency room, buy new equipment, hire Dr. Huntington away from the University. Yet when the mayor was brought here, the key ingredient, physicians sufficiently experienced in trauma to save the mayor's life, were not available. And according to Dr. Huntington you do not have the support of most of the staff in this venture to set up a trauma center."

"Mrs. Normans, building staff support takes time."

"How much time, Mr. Anthony? Six months? A year? Two years? How many deaths are we to be responsible for in the meantime?"

He felt now that he was on the run, the snapping at his heels coming closer and closer.

"I'm sorry. We had to start somewhere, Mrs. Normans. I was convinced, and still am, that if I can prove to our staff that the trauma center could bring in patients, they'll ultimately come around to the idea of supporting our effort."

Marden, impatience showing on his face, took over. "Enough is enough. Al, we have talked matters over and have come to several conclusions. First, this hospital is going to pull back from its efforts to gain de facto recognition as a trauma center. At this point I would doubt that we would even submit an application if the county follows Dr. Kirk's advice to establish a bidding process.

But perhaps more important, the board has decided that it is no longer in Coit Hill's interests to have you serve as its chief administrator."

Anthony paled. "But—"

"I'm sorry, Al, but there can be no backing away from that decision. The hospital will be subject to tremendous legal and community pressures as a result of your actions and, to be plain, removing you from the post is one clear signal that we mean to change direction."

"Mr. Marden . . ."

"You will remain on our payroll for two months while you look for another position. The hospital will also assume whatever legal costs you are likely to have as a result of the events surrounding the mayor. But as of five P.M. this afternoon you are relieved of your duties."

Anthony looked around the table, hoping someone would speak up, someone would suggest that perhaps there was a better way, that after all the hard work he had done for the hospital, he should be given a second chance. No one spoke.

"Al," Marden finally said. "If you'll excuse us?"

Anthony slowly pushed his chair back and rose. He started to pick up the folders he had brought with him, but changed his mind. Stepping sideways, he squeezed out from between the chair and table. In three more steps he was out the door. As he walked slowly away, he could hear the muffled voices as the board resumed its discussion behind the door that he had closed behind him.

17

Allan was drying himself off, vigorously slapping the big towel over his body, when Julie came into the bathroom carrying two mugs of coffee.

She handed him one. "Three spoons of sugar enough?" she asked.

He took a sip and grimaced. "More than enough. I've got so much adrenaline pounding through me I could fly to work."

"Are you nervous about it?"

"I'd say. It's been months since I operated on anyone. Skills degenerate fast. That and, well, the environment." He slipped into his briefs, then combed his hair.

"You're worried about the welcome you'll get from the trauma team? What on earth for? It's just Santorre, Fedder, and the rest. They've been on your side all along."

"I'm not worried about them," Allan answered. "It's Dorr and the others. Just the fact that they've conveniently arranged for me to work the graveyard shift my first day back on the job is indicative of their attitude."

Julie watched him lather his face with quick circular motions, then winced as he moved the straight-edged razor he favored over his face. "Pardon the French, but fuck 'em and the white horse they rode in on," she said.

"Easy for you to say. But Steinhardt, you know, carved Dorr and White each a new asshole in the process of getting me reinstated. I've been a lot of aggravation to them. There are deep scars that will take a long time to heal over."

With half a dozen quick strokes he was finished. He rinsed his face, then leaned forward to inspect himself closely in the mirror. Satisfied, he doused himself with after-shave lotion. He let out a little whimper of pain as the liquid braced his skin.

Julie stepped back into the bedroom. He followed her and, with a flick of his wrist, plucked a pair of pants off the bed.

"Allan, try not to let them upset you."

He buckled the belt, then studied her. "It's a promise," he said. He searched her face. "Julie, I have the feeling that something's bothering you."

She shook her head.

"Come on, girl. You've been acting a bit funny the last few days. A bit far away."

She sat down on the edge of his bed. He followed and sat next to her. "Julie?"

"I don't know, Allan. I'm not even sure I can put it into words."

"Well, you'd better try, because I'm not leaving here until I know what's eating you."

Julie turned around, put her arms around him, and pressed her forehead to his neck.

He held her for a moment, then pushed her back.

"Julie, what is it?"

Her eyes moistened. "Since things started going your way, Allan, you've grown distant too. Now that you're on the offensive, you're growing progressively preoccupied. Whenever you are around here, you're on the phone with Younger or Creighton or Steinhardt. And when you're not on the phone, you're dashing out to a meeting with them or someone else. And when you're not with them or talking to your advisers, you sit on that couch, withdrawn."

He caressed her cheek. "Julie, I care a lot about you, I love you. Being with you, having you support me, made me realize, for the first time in my life, how awfully lonely life could be without you. You were there. You were the only one who stood by me, who gave me some hope. But Julie, it's not that I'm keeping things in. It's that I'm still not in the clear. It may look to you like I'm on the offensive, but I may go back to the hospital and find out that people have lost residencies because of me. My research is in pieces and I have no idea how to start putting it back together again. And I still don't have a clear idea of where the trauma fight is going to wind up. As much as I want to, I can't say to you: this is it, let's commit to each other now and forever. I'm not sure I have the right to do that just yet."

"I wasn't asking for an eternal commitment. But I don't want a part-time relationship either, one in which you don't share your thoughts. I don't want to be a superficial part of your life. That's all I was trying to say."

She rose and walked away. He went to the dresser and took a shirt out of a drawer. He put it on, buttoned it, and tucked it into his pants, aware that Julie was watching him from the other side of the room. "Julie . . ."

"It's all right, Allan," she said quietly. "When is this shift over for you?"

"A long twenty-four hours from now."

There was room for his car closer to the emergency-room entrance, but he parked as far away as possible on purpose. He had told Julie that he was not worried about the reception he would get from his colleagues, but within himself he was not so sure. He was apprehensive, nervous, even scared. The long walk to the emergency room would give him time to calm down. He wanted to walk in as if nothing untoward had happened, as if he were coming back after having gone home after his last shift to catch a few hours of sleep.

As soon as the automatic doors started to pull apart to allow him to pass, the clapping and the cheers began. The welcome was coming from Santorre, Fedder, Maggie, several other residents and interns, nurses who worked the emergency room, and many he knew who were assigned to services on other floors. An old bed sheet had been improvised into a "WELCOME BACK, ALLAN" banner that had been draped above the nurse's station. The top of the counter had been cleared of its usual clutter of paperwork to make room for a huge cake molded to resemble a bedpan. There was a punch bowl brimming with a pink liquid. Paper partyware was neatly arrayed on both sides of the cake.

"It's a good thing you're coming back on a Monday night," Maggie said, stepping forward. "We've only got two or three people out there bleeding to death, so we have time for a little party." She warmly embraced him.

Allan wanted to protest, but squelched the thought—though the effort to keep his eyes from watering was not nearly as successful. Fedder, aware that Allan was struggling with his emotions, came over, threw an arm around his shoulders, and led him to the counter. "Schmuck!" he said as they walked. "You have any idea how we've been busting ass while you were gone?"

Allan opened his mouth, hoping something witty would come out. No words emerged. Fedder laughed and began to cut the cake, giving Allan the first piece, then handing out other portions to the welcoming party. "Well, never mind," Fedder went on. "We took a vote and decided that as your punishment Brooks is going to do all your cut-downs for you for the next month." There was good-natured laughter, including a guffaw from Maggie who, having grown proficient at the procedure, stuck her tongue out at Fedder.

They stood and talked, everyone, particularly Allan, working hard to keep the conversation from straying into troublesome ground. To Allan's profound relief the screams of a siren cut through the conversation and the jokes. Though the nurses and residents who had come down from other floors calmly went on sipping, eating, and chatting, Allan, Santorre, Fedder, and Maggie, almost in unison, dropped their plates into a trash can and ran toward the ambulance entrance.

A van, which they immediately recognized as the vehicle that sometimes brought prisoners from San Quentin, pulled a bit past the entrance, then made a fast backward U-turn until its back doors were two feet from where Allan and the others were standing.

"Got a G.I. bleeder here," the driver said as he jumped out of the front seat and headed to the back of the van.

"A cirrhotic?" Santorre asked as he helped open the door and reached in to draw out the stretcher. Another man, a prison guard, also emerged from the back of the van.

"Nah, don't think so," the guard answered as he and the driver helped Fedder and Allan place the convict on the gurney and propel him inside. "He's not an old alkie."

Allan, who through the party had felt vague waves of apprehension still moving through him, suddenly realized the doubts had evaporated and began barking out his orders in quick and clipped fashion. IVs, saline solutions, tubes, lavage trays, a portable X-ray machine materialized around the convict's bed.

They cut the man's clothes off and even before his pants had fallen to the floor, Allan was running his hands over the patient's chest and abdomen. There were no signs that the man had been stabbed or shot.

"Was he in a fight that you know of?" Allan asked the guard.

"Nah. Everything was quiet till his cellmate started screaming for us. What we got out of him was that this guy's been vomiting for a couple of days. But tonight he started barfin' blood. That's when he called us."

"His blood pressure is a little low, 70/50," Maggie said after she had inserted an IV and began to release fluids into the man's vein. "What do you think is going on?" Maggie asked.

"I don't know, but whatever it is, he isn't trauma-center material. But we might as well take a look at him, nothing else is going on." Allan stared down at the man, then addressed him directly. "What's going on, buddy? Where do you hurt?"

"My stomach, man."

"You ever have any trouble with it before?"

"Got me an ulcer, you know. But it's never been this bad."

Allan contemplated him for a moment, then turned to Maggie. "Let's get a portable abdominal X ray and the routine blood work."

"Hey, man," the con yelled. "I don't need no X rays. Don't want to be exposed to that stuff. Just give me some medicine for the ulcers, that's all I need."

"I don't think so, fella," Allan said. "No X rays, no medicine."

A technician and a resident pushed the portable X-ray machine over to the bed and positioned it over the patient. Allan, Maggie, Fedder, and the other residents and nurses backed twenty feet away from the bed. There was the familiar whirr of the machine going into action. As soon as the sound had faded and the technician had his film, they all moved back. Five minutes later the technician returned.

Allan took the X-ray film and pushed it into the light box near the convict's bed. When he flicked the button to turn on the light, Fedder snickered almost as soon as the details of the black and white picture sprang into view. Maggie leaned closer. "What the hell are all those things in his stomach?"

"Take another look," Allan said. She put her face to within inches of the X ray, then turned around, astounded, to face Allan. "Razor blades? You mean to tell me that man has three razor blades in his stomach?"

"That's what they are, doc," the guard said. "Razor blades."

"But . . ." She was too dumbfounded to say more.

"The guy probably had a score to settle with someone," the guard went on. "Probably wanted to go after someone's ass."

"But why swallow them himself?" Maggie was fascinated.

"Because that's how he got them into the prison. Old trick. He has his old lady bring him razor blades. His old lady covers the razors with tape and keeps them in her mouth. When she kisses him, she passes them into his mouth and he swallows them. Next time he takes a crap, they come out. The next day he has a weapon to cut someone's throat."

"Well, this one either wasn't too lucky or his old lady didn't know how to wrap razors," Allan interrupted. "Given his history of ulcers, I would say he's got some scarring and narrowing of the channel leading from the stomach to the duodenum. The wrapping from the razor blades probably plugged it off completely and whatever food or water he was taking in backed up into his stomach." Allan pointed to the X ray. "You can see how distended the stomach is."

"Do we take him into surgery?" Maggie asked.

Allan looked over at the convict, who was lying back, disgust etched all over his face. "Not immediately. Let's put a tube down and drain his stomach, give him some IVs and admit him. But I would say that in the next couple of days he is going to need surgery."

"Waste of the taxpayer's money if you ask me, doc," the guard chimed in. "Fucker shoulda sucked gas ten years ago."

"Not exactly a sterling trauma case to welcome you back," Santorre said to Allan as they walked away.

Allan smiled. "At this point I'd treat a hangnail just to get my hands on a patient again."

They walked to the floor that had been set aside for trauma victims who had been released from the intensive-care unit but who still needed specialized attention. Santorre stopped in front of the second room to the left of the nurses' station and quietly opened the door. There were two men in the room, both sound asleep. Santorre walked back to the nurses' station and picked up their charts. Allan, meanwhile, walked into the room, looked both men over, and squinted at the blood pressure and heart monitor machines over their beds.

"The patient on the left is the kid that lost his legs in that freak accident with the elevator cable," Santorre whispered. "He's doing very well. He's accepted the loss of the legs and has really gotten into physical therapy. We've even had to slow him down some because he was overexerting himself. But it's not an entirely happy ending."

"Because of the old man?"

"In a way. The brother just went to pieces because he

couldn't save the old man too. Had a nervous breakdown about three weeks ago. He came through the E.R. with a stomach full of tranquilizers. We just barely pulled him through."

"Is he in the psych ward here?"

"We found him a bed for a couple of days but then transferred him up the hill to Langley-Porter."

"The guy on the right," Santorre whispered, "is our jogger. We took out the tracheal tube three days ago. The lab tests are showing continued improvement in kidney function. I think we can take out the Scribner shunt over the weekend and get him off dialysis. We plan on starting him on an oral diet Monday or Tuesday."

"How about his physical therapy?"

"Making progress there too. They think he's about ready to start walking on his own."

"How's his wife doing?"

"Not bad. Great, in fact. Maggie said she walked in on them the other day, before we moved this other guy in, and he had his hand up his wife's skirt."

"I don't know why we bother with lab tests," Allan said. "The best sign of recovery is the first sign of horniness."

The jogger, who had been sleeping with his back to them, stirred and turned around. He switched on the lamp above his bed and sat up. "What'a going on?" he whispered. "What time is it?"

"Sorry," Santorre said, stepping closer to the bed. "Two o'clock. Dr. Kirk is back on duty and I was just bringing him up to speed."

The jogger looked past Santorre. "Dr. Kirk? The guy that operated on me? Goddamn, I've been wanting to meet you. Doctor, whatever you ever need or want . . ."

Allan came forward. "Don't think about it. It's just nice to see you doing so well."

The jogger smiled. "Say, you guys know of anyone on this floor who could use a dozen long-stemmed roses? This is the third bunch the people at the office have sent. There's somebody around here who has to need them more."

"Thanks, I'm sure there is," Santorre said. "I'll ask around. Get back to sleep. We'll check back in the morning."

Santorre and Allan wandered slowly to the vending-machine nook near the emergency room.

"What's happening with you these last few days?" Santorre asked. "We hear you're making a lot of speeches around town."

"Morning, noon, and night. Steinhardt believes that a good offense is the better part of valor, not to mention a good defense."

"Do you think that's why you got reinstated?"

Allan shook his head. "I got reinstated because Steinhardt threatened the University with all kinds of court actions unless they put me back on pending some formal hearings. No, he thinks the more I talk about trauma care publicly, the less I'll look like some crazy who's doing Transylvanian experiments here."

"And you agree with him?"

"In part. I don't think it'll get me back to where I was before all this started, but it may help. But I am hoping the talking will help keep the trauma issue from cooling down."

"And what about your other . . ."

"Troubles?"

"Yeah."

"Steinhardt's scenario is this. He thinks we should fight all the lawsuits and not even talk about settling. NIH, he says, will bar me from receiving federal research funds for at least two years. The University will go through a bunch of rigmarole to make it look as if they are giving me due process, then formally relieve me of my duties as chairman of the new trauma surgery section and will limit me to do research only under the supervision of a senior scientist. But Steinhardt thinks they'll let me keep my standing as an assistant professor of surgery, which means that I can go on working as a surgeon here."

"And what about the Board of Medical Quality Assurance? Are they going to move on your license?"

"Steinhardt thinks they might have nailed me if I were still really low, but now that I'm looking good they'll just ignore me."

"What makes him so sure?"

"Steinhardt has had dealings with them. They go after the drug abusers, which is okay. But in terms of docs who screw up medically, Bumqua grandstands by landing on some poor slob who has missed a diagnosis of some obscure condition in a four-A.M. consult. But they ignore the butcher who is killing patients but has a lot of legal clout."

"You think they are putting you in that category?"

"Well, not in the butcher category. But in the group that has sufficient legal help to make them think twice about devoting their meager bureaucratic resources to a fight they'll not likely win. They'll be glad to let the complaint against me gather dust."

"You going to go on with that subcommittee the Joint Committee asked you to head?"

"Sure. Why not? Nobody's doubted my dedication to trauma care."

"I guess not. But I'll tell you one thing. We all sure hope you can get that subcommittee in gear and get things going because it's been sheer hell around here," Santorre said as they sat down on a bench near one of the vending machines. Here it comes, Allan thought. There was resentment against him among his trauma-team colleagues after all. He took a deep breath. "Look, I'm sorry if my troubles with the University have caused you all problems."

"They haven't caused us problems, Allan. We've been with you all the way. If you had let us help, we would have."

Allan was puzzled. "Then what? Is it that my suspension meant you were shorthanded?"

"No, your suspension wasn't what caused us problems either. First, I do think that crazy idea of yours about a boycott did have some impact. We did start seeing an increase in our volume right after that. Then when Anthony got the ax and Coit Hill closed down their trauma operation, we started getting even more cases. People who were barely conscious after accidents were begging to be brought here, relatives of trauma patients started demanding that their loved ones be rushed here. We've even had a couple of cases where people had scribbled instructions on their insurance cards for them to be brought here in case of an emergency. Either everybody decided that if things were a mess at Coit Hill, they had to be just as bad at other community hospitals, or they just simply carried your call for a boycott one step further and started to bring their business here. There were days when we ran out of intensive-care beds and had to shift patients out earlier than we would have wanted to. I mean, it's been bedlam."

"Has Dorr tried to help out?"

"Yeah, he's tried, but it's been tough on him too. We've had a couple of real set-to's because daytime trauma cases have bumped cancer and heart patients from the surgery schedule. A couple of oncology surgeons and cardiac guys have raised holy hell. I hear that it got to the point where one of the cardiac surgeons threatened to leave the hospital. It's been a real mess."

"Joe. What are you driving at? You saying I shouldn't have talked out about trauma? That I shouldn't have focused attention on us?"

"No, we all know you had to do it, Allan. But the thing is that we have become the de facto trauma center for the city and we can't work that way. If we are going to take more trauma cases, then we should have a formal designation so that we can make it work properly. We need to organize the transport system so that paramedics aren't making medical decisions by themselves, so that the good citizens of this community understand who comes to a trauma center and who doesn't. Most of all we need to get community hospitals to agree formally to give up trauma cases so that we can do some planning about the numbers of people we can expect. What I'm saying is that we need to organize this thing or it will drive us crazy at best or still leave people dying unnecessarily at worst."

"So what exactly are you asking me to do?"

"Ram a plan through the Board of Supervisors. This thing just can't go at the usual snail's pace at which the county makes decisions."

Allan stood up and walked to the hot-drink machine in the corner of the lounge. According to the red lights beneath the machine's buttons, the only remaining drink that could be bought was chicken-flavored soup. Allan put a quarter in the slot and gave the soup button a sharp jab. A cup dropped to the bottom of the opening through which the drinks were dispensed but came to rest at an angle. As Allan reached in to straighten out the cup, the machine began to pour out its version of chicken soup. Half of the steaming liquid landed on his hand, the rest in the cup. When the machine stopped, he took out the half-empty cup, then gave the machine a vicious kick.

"Jesus, I hate these things," he muttered, then turned back to Santorre. "Joe, listen. You know I can't do that. In the first place, I can't make it seem as though all I've wanted to do was involve this hospital in a power struggle with Anthony and that all I was interested in was my own glory. In the second place, and more important, there has to be a rational designation process and every hospital that wants it has to have a shot at the designation or they just won't buy into the concept at all."

"Then what are the chances that one of those other hospitals will get it?"

"Realistically? Slim to none. Not because I intend to fix it, but because I would say that no one can commit to trauma as we have done. We have most of the resources, especially in that we have the people and are fully staffed twenty-four hours a day. In spite of some bitching, we do have the backing of a lot of our docs. Even if the other hospital administrators try to go for the designation more honorably than Anthony, they will still have to go out and sell their staffs on the idea, not to mention their boards. And if Coit Hill couldn't do all that without resorting to some underhanded tactics, I doubt that any other hospital in this area could."

"Fine, but if we do get the designation, don't think you're off the hook. You still are going to have to be the one to make sure that we get to do it right."

"Meaning?"

"Meaning that since we are in part county funded, the people downtown will expect us to pull off miracles without adding penny one to our budget. Even if we are not an independent department anymore, the leadership is still on you. You're going to have to fight for us as hard as you have fought for your trauma victims. Otherwise, don't expect much help from us. We like you and love to work with you, Allan. But we're not crazy. There are cushy jobs in trauma opening up around the country. And having trained here it wouldn't be too hard for any one of us to find one of those jobs if you start jacking us around by asking us to work our asses off without the benefit of some good additional support. I hate to be that blunt, but someone has to tell you."

Allan took a long drink of soup. "Okay. I wouldn't trust you if I didn't think you could be honest when you had to be." He looked down into his cup, studying the sediment in the remaining watery liquid.

"Hey, where'd you drift off to?" Santorre asked. "What are you thinking about?"

Allan flashed a generous smile. "That maybe you'd better get somebody to cover for me for a couple of hours."

"Are you nuts? Where are you going?"

"Got to go see Julie. Be back in two hours. Tops."

"Kirk, you off on another of your impulsive moves?"

Without answering, Allan dashed back to the jogger's room. Allan slowly opened the door and peered in. Only the sound of soft snoring greeted him. He slowly made his way to the dresser at the side of the room and scooped up the vase with the roses.

Fifteen minutes later he was bending over Julie, softly kissing the nape of her neck. She stirred, turned over and opened her eyes. "Allan?"

He switched on the bedside lamp. Julie pressed her eyes together. When she opened them her gaze fell on the flowers. "Where did you get roses at four in the morning?"

"Never mind that." He took her face in his hands and brought her closer to him. Her eyes stayed open even as she felt his lips touch hers. When he drew back, her gaze was still on him.

"Julie, I guess I'm just plain dumb, and it takes me a little while to figure some things out. I love you, Julie. I'm going to need all the love and support you can give me."

"Allan . . ."

"Shhh. Listen. I realize that I was withdrawing from you when I was running around and planning things without filling you in. I was taking you for granted. But I'm not going to do that to you again, Julie. Ever." He leaned forward and kissed her.

Julie pulled back a bit. "You going back to the hospital?"

"I told Santorre I'd be back in a couple of hours. I still have an hour and fifteen minutes."

"Time enough to fool around a little bit."

"And maybe talk about when we could get away to get married?"

"Possibly," Julie said, laughing. "Possibly."

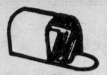

FREE!!
BOOKS BY MAIL
CATALOGUE

BOOKS BY MAIL will share with you our current bestselling books as well as hard to find specialty titles in areas that will match your interests. You will be updated on what's new in books at no cost to you. Just fill in the coupon below and discover the convenience of having books delivered to your home.

PLEASE ADD $1.00 TO COVER THE COST OF POSTAGE & HANDLING.

- -

BOOKS BY MAIL

320 Steelcase Road E.,
Markham, Ontario L3R 2M1

IN THE U.S. -
210 5th Ave., 7th Floor
New York, N.Y., 10010

Please send Books By Mail catalogue to:

Name _____
(please print)

Address _____

City _____

Prov./State _____ P.C./Zip _____

(BBM1)